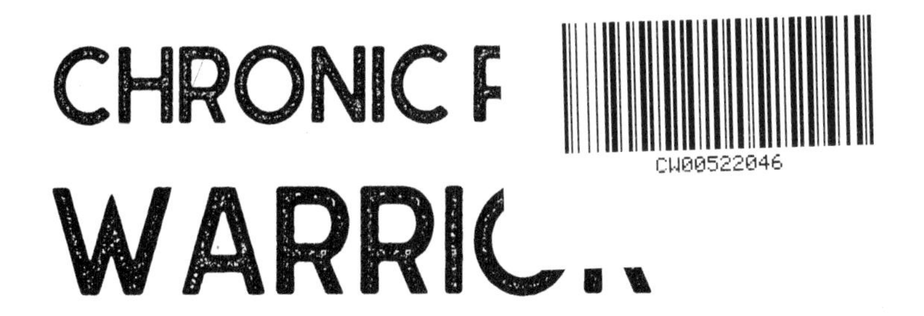

A pain & symptom tracking journal

WELLNESS WARRIOR PRESS
www.wellnesswarriorpress.com

ISBN: 9798721938634

This journal belongs to...

STU (EBANEEZAGONE) JECKELL

DOCTOR / SPECIALIST INFORMATION

Name	Address	Contact

DAILY MEDICATION / SUPPLEMENTS

Medication / Supplement	Dosage

SUMMARY

For each journal entry, return to this summary page and rate your overall pain / discomfort level (1 being no pain and 10 being unbearable)

Entry #	Rating	Entry #	Rating
1		31	
2		32	
3		33	
4		34	
5		35	
6		36	
7		37	
8		38	
9		39	
10		40	
11		41	
12		42	
13		43	
14		44	
15		45	
16		46	
17		47	
18		48	
19		49	
20		50	
21		51	
22		52	
23		53	
24		54	
25		55	
26		56	
27		57	
28		58	
29		59	
30		60	

Date: April 18th 2022

HOW ARE YOU FEELING TODAY?

Like death

Terrible

Not good

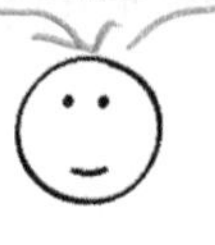
Meh

Good

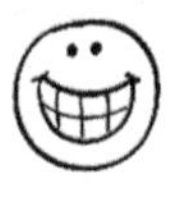
Great!

Amazing!

RATE YOUR PAIN LEVEL

1 2 3 4 5 6 7 8 9 10

Describe your pain / symptoms — Where do you feel it?

	am	pm
Lower back	☒	☒
Shoulder	☐	☒
finger	☐	☒
heels	☒	☒
Ebow	☒	☒
	☐	☐
	☐	☐
	☐	☐

Front *Back*

What about your...?

Mood	1 2 3 4 5 6 7 8 9 10
Energy levels	1 2 3 4 5 6 7 8 9 10
Mental clarity	1 2 3 4 5 6 7 8 9 10

Feeling sick?

- ☐ Nope!
- ☐ Yes...

- ☐ Nausea
- ☐ Diarrhea
- ☐ Vomiting
- ☐ Sore throat
- ☐ Congestion
- ☐ Coughing
- ☐ Chills
- ☐ Fever

Other symptoms: ____________

LET'S EXPLORE SOME MORE

#1

Hours of Sleep	1	2	3	4	5	6	7	8	9	10	+
Sleep Quality	1	2	3	4	5	6	7	8	9	10	

WEATHER

☐ Hot ☐ Mild ☐ Cold BM Pressure: ____

☐ Dry ☐ Humid ☐ Wet Allergen Levels: ____

STRESS LEVELS

None	Low	Medium	High	Max	@$#%!

FOOD / MEDICATIONS

FOOD / DRINKS

MEDS / SUPPLEMENTS	TIME	DOSE

☐ usual daily medication

EXERCISE / DAILY ACTIVITY

☐ Heck yes, I worked out.

☐ I managed to exercise a bit.

☐ No, I haven't exercised at all.

☐ I did some stuff, and that counts.

DETAILS

NOTES / TRIGGERS / IMPROVEMENTS

WRITE ONE THING YOU'RE GRATEFUL FOR

Date: April 19 2022

HOW ARE YOU FEELING TODAY?

					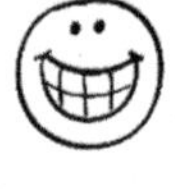	
Like death	Terrible	Not good	Meh	Good ✓	Great!	Amazing!

RATE YOUR PAIN LEVEL

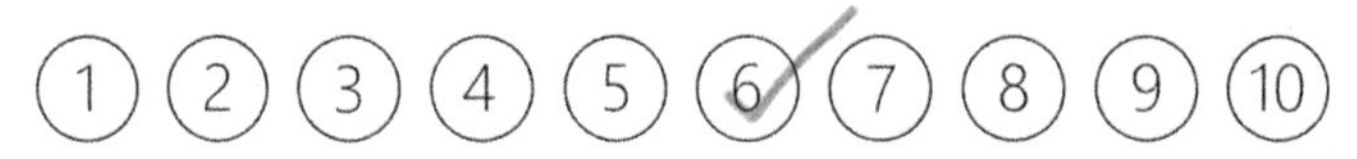

Pain level marked: 6

Describe your pain / symptoms	am	pm
lower back	☐	☐
heels	☐	☐
knees	☐	☐
shoulder	☐	☐
	☐	☐
	☐	☐
	☐	☐
	☐	☐

Where do you feel it? Front / Back

What about your...?

	1	2	3	4	5	6	7	8	9	10
Mood						✓				
Energy levels							✓			
Mental clarity						✓				

Feeling sick?

- ☑ Nope!
- ☐ Yes...

- ☐ Nausea
- ☐ Diarrhea
- ☐ Vomiting
- ☐ Sore throat
- ☐ Congestion
- ☐ Coughing
- ☐ Chills
- ☐ Fever

Other symptoms: ____

LET'S EXPLORE SOME MORE #2

Hours of Sleep	1	2	3	4 (filled)	5	6	7	8	9	10	+
Sleep Quality	1	2	3	4	5 (filled)	6	7	8	9	10	

(5) From 11 am to 4 pm

WEATHER

- [ ] Hot
- [x] Mild
- [ ] Cold
- BM Pressure: ______
- [ ] Dry
- [ ] Humid
- [ ] Wet
- Allergen Levels: ______

STRESS LEVELS

None | **(Low)** | Medium | High | Max | @$#%!

FOOD / MEDICATIONS

FOOD / DRINKS	MEDS / SUPPLEMENTS	TIME	DOSE
Tuna Salad 5 slices of cheese			
Pinapple chunks			
lucozade Red pepper 1/2			
McDonalds hash			
brown. 1/4 cucumber			
Double sausage			
McMuffin coffee			

- [ ] usual daily medication

EXERCISE / DAILY ACTIVITY

- [ ] Heck yes, I worked out.
- [x] I managed to exercise a bit.
- [ ] No, I haven't exercised at all.
- [ ] I did some stuff, and that counts.

DETAILS

NOTES / TRIGGERS / IMPROVEMENTS

WRITE ONE THING YOU'RE GRATEFUL FOR

Date: ______________

HOW ARE YOU FEELING TODAY?

Like death	Terrible	Not good	Meh	Good	Great!	Amazing!

RATE YOUR PAIN LEVEL

1 2 3 4 5 6 7 8 9 10

Describe your pain / symptoms	am	pm
	☐	☐
	☐	☐
	☐	☐
	☐	☐
	☐	☐
	☐	☐
	☐	☐
	☐	☐

Where do you feel it?

Front *Back*

What about your...?

Mood	1	2	3	4	5	6	7	8	9	10
Energy levels	1	2	3	4	5	6	7	8	9	10
Mental clarity	1	2	3	4	5	6	7	8	9	10

Feeling sick?

☐ Nope!
☐ Yes...

☐ Nausea ☐ Diarrhea ☐ Vomiting ☐ Sore throat
☐ Congestion ☐ Coughing ☐ Chills ☐ Fever

Other symptoms: ______________________

LET'S EXPLORE SOME MORE #3

Hours of Sleep	1 2 3 4 5 6 7 8 9 10 +
Sleep Quality	1 2 3 4 5 6 7 8 9 10

WEATHER

- ☐ Hot ☐ Mild ☐ Cold BM Pressure: ______
- ☐ Dry ☐ Humid ☐ Wet Allergen Levels: ______

STRESS LEVELS

None	Low	Medium	High	Max	@$#%!

FOOD / MEDICATIONS

FOOD / DRINKS

MEDS / SUPPLEMENTS	TIME	DOSE

☐ usual daily medication

EXERCISE / DAILY ACTIVITY

- ☐ Heck yes, I worked out.
- ☐ I managed to exercise a bit.
- ☐ No, I haven't exercised at all.
- ☐ I did some stuff, and that counts.

DETAILS

NOTES / TRIGGERS / IMPROVEMENTS

WRITE ONE THING YOU'RE GRATEFUL FOR

Date: ______________

HOW ARE YOU FEELING TODAY?

     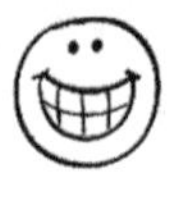 

Like death	Terrible	Not good	Meh	Good	Great!	Amazing!

RATE YOUR PAIN LEVEL

① ② ③ ④ ⑤ ⑥ ⑦ ⑧ ⑨ ⑩

Describe your pain / symptoms	am	pm
	☐	☐
	☐	☐
	☐	☐
	☐	☐
	☐	☐
	☐	☐
	☐	☐
	☐	☐

Where do you feel it?

Front *Back*

What about your...?

Mood	1 2 3 4 5 6 7 8 9 10
Energy levels	1 2 3 4 5 6 7 8 9 10
Mental clarity	1 2 3 4 5 6 7 8 9 10

Feeling sick?

☐ Nope!
☐ Yes...

☐ Nausea ☐ Diarrhea ☐ Vomiting ☐ Sore throat
☐ Congestion ☐ Coughing ☐ Chills ☐ Fever

Other symptoms: ______________________________

LET'S EXPLORE SOME MORE #4

Hours of Sleep	1	2	3	4	5	6	7	8	9	10	+
Sleep Quality	1	2	3	4	5	6	7	8	9	10	

WEATHER

- [ ] Hot
- [ ] Mild
- [ ] Cold
- [ ] Dry
- [ ] Humid
- [ ] Wet

BM Pressure: ____

Allergen Levels: ____

STRESS LEVELS

None	Low	Medium	High	Max	@$#%!

FOOD / MEDICATIONS

FOOD / DRINKS

MEDS / SUPPLEMENTS	TIME	DOSE

- [ ] usual daily medication

EXERCISE / DAILY ACTIVITY

- [ ] Heck yes, I worked out.
- [ ] I managed to exercise a bit.
- [ ] No, I haven't exercised at all.
- [ ] I did some stuff, and that counts.

DETAILS

NOTES / TRIGGERS / IMPROVEMENTS

WRITE ONE THING YOU'RE GRATEFUL FOR

*Date:*______________

HOW ARE YOU FEELING TODAY?

 Like death

 Terrible

 Not good

 Meh

 Good

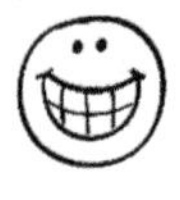 Great!

 Amazing!

RATE YOUR PAIN LEVEL

① ② ③ ④ ⑤ ⑥ ⑦ ⑧ ⑨ ⑩

Describe your pain / symptoms	am	pm
	☐	☐
	☐	☐
	☐	☐
	☐	☐
	☐	☐
	☐	☐
	☐	☐
	☐	☐

Where do you feel it?

Front *Back*

What about your...?

Mood	① ② ③ ④ ⑤ ⑥ ⑦ ⑧ ⑨ ⑩
Energy levels	① ② ③ ④ ⑤ ⑥ ⑦ ⑧ ⑨ ⑩
Mental clarity	① ② ③ ④ ⑤ ⑥ ⑦ ⑧ ⑨ ⑩

Feeling sick?

☐ Nope!

☐ Yes...

☐ Nausea ☐ Diarrhea ☐ Vomiting ☐ Sore throat

☐ Congestion ☐ Coughing ☐ Chills ☐ Fever

Other symptoms: ______________________________

LET'S EXPLORE SOME MORE

Hours of Sleep	1	2	3	4	5	6	7	8	9	10	+
Sleep Quality	1	2	3	4	5	6	7	8	9	10	

WEATHER

- ☐ Hot ☐ Mild ☐ Cold BM Pressure: ____
- ☐ Dry ☐ Humid ☐ Wet Allergen Levels: ____

STRESS LEVELS

None	Low	Medium	High	Max	@$#%!

FOOD / MEDICATIONS

FOOD / DRINKS

MEDS / SUPPLEMENTS	TIME	DOSE

☐ usual daily medication

EXERCISE / DAILY ACTIVITY

- ☐ Heck yes, I worked out.
- ☐ I managed to exercise a bit.
- ☐ No, I haven't exercised at all.
- ☐ I did some stuff, and that counts.

DETAILS

NOTES / TRIGGERS / IMPROVEMENTS

WRITE ONE THING YOU'RE GRATEFUL FOR

Date: ______________

HOW ARE YOU FEELING TODAY?

Like death	Terrible	Not good	Meh	Good	Great!	Amazing!

RATE YOUR PAIN LEVEL

① ② ③ ④ ⑤ ⑥ ⑦ ⑧ ⑨ ⑩

Describe your pain / symptoms	am	pm
	☐	☐
	☐	☐
	☐	☐
	☐	☐
	☐	☐
	☐	☐
	☐	☐
	☐	☐

Where do you feel it?

Front *Back*

What about your...?

Mood	① ② ③ ④ ⑤ ⑥ ⑦ ⑧ ⑨ ⑩
Energy levels	① ② ③ ④ ⑤ ⑥ ⑦ ⑧ ⑨ ⑩
Mental clarity	① ② ③ ④ ⑤ ⑥ ⑦ ⑧ ⑨ ⑩

Feeling sick?

☐ Nope!

☐ Yes...

☐ Nausea	☐ Diarrhea	☐ Vomiting	☐ Sore throat
☐ Congestion	☐ Coughing	☐ Chills	☐ Fever

Other symptoms: ______________________________

LET'S EXPLORE SOME MORE #6

Hours of Sleep	1 2 3 4 5 6 7 8 9 10 +
Sleep Quality	1 2 3 4 5 6 7 8 9 10

WEATHER

☐ Hot ☐ Mild ☐ Cold BM Pressure: ______

☐ Dry ☐ Humid ☐ Wet Allergen Levels: ______

STRESS LEVELS

None	Low	Medium	High	Max	@$#%!

FOOD / MEDICATIONS

FOOD / DRINKS

MEDS / SUPPLEMENTS	TIME	DOSE

☐ usual daily medication

EXERCISE / DAILY ACTIVITY

☐ Heck yes, I worked out.

☐ I managed to exercise a bit.

☐ No, I haven't exercised at all.

☐ I did some stuff, and that counts.

DETAILS

NOTES / TRIGGERS / IMPROVEMENTS

WRITE ONE THING YOU'RE GRATEFUL FOR

*Date:*______________

HOW ARE YOU FEELING TODAY?

     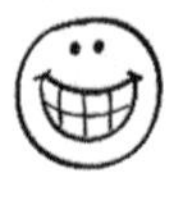 

Like death	Terrible	Not good	Meh	Good	Great!	Amazing!

RATE YOUR PAIN LEVEL

① ② ③ ④ ⑤ ⑥ ⑦ ⑧ ⑨ ⑩

Describe your pain / symptoms	am	pm
	☐	☐
	☐	☐
	☐	☐
	☐	☐
	☐	☐
	☐	☐
	☐	☐
	☐	☐

Where do you feel it?

Front *Back*

What about your...?

Mood	① ② ③ ④ ⑤ ⑥ ⑦ ⑧ ⑨ ⑩
Energy levels	① ② ③ ④ ⑤ ⑥ ⑦ ⑧ ⑨ ⑩
Mental clarity	① ② ③ ④ ⑤ ⑥ ⑦ ⑧ ⑨ ⑩

Feeling sick?

☐ Nope!
☐ Yes...

☐ Nausea	☐ Diarrhea	☐ Vomiting	☐ Sore throat
☐ Congestion	☐ Coughing	☐ Chills	☐ Fever

Other symptoms: ______________________________

LET'S EXPLORE SOME MORE

#7

Hours of Sleep	1 2 3 4 5 6 7 8 9 10 +
Sleep Quality	1 2 3 4 5 6 7 8 9 10

WEATHER

- ☐ Hot ☐ Mild ☐ Cold BM Pressure: ____
- ☐ Dry ☐ Humid ☐ Wet Allergen Levels: ____

STRESS LEVELS

None Low Medium High Max @$#%!

FOOD / MEDICATIONS

FOOD / DRINKS

MEDS / SUPPLEMENTS	TIME	DOSE

☐ usual daily medication

EXERCISE / DAILY ACTIVITY

- ☐ Heck yes, I worked out.
- ☐ I managed to exercise a bit.
- ☐ No, I haven't exercised at all.
- ☐ I did some stuff, and that counts.

DETAILS

NOTES / TRIGGERS / IMPROVEMENTS

WRITE ONE THING YOU'RE GRATEFUL FOR

Date: ______________

HOW ARE YOU FEELING TODAY?

     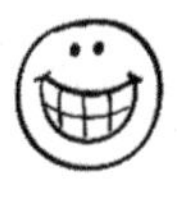 

Like death	Terrible	Not good	Meh	Good	Great!	Amazing!

RATE YOUR PAIN LEVEL

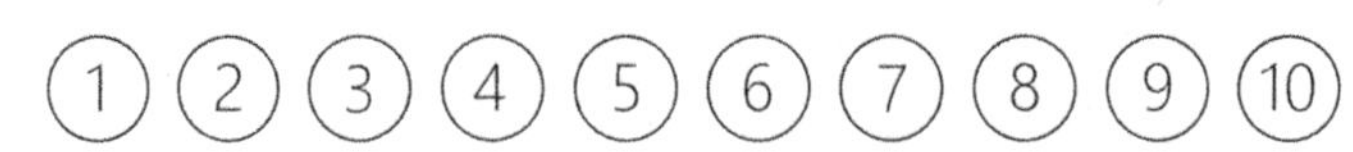

Describe your pain / symptoms

	am	pm
	☐	☐
	☐	☐
	☐	☐
	☐	☐
	☐	☐
	☐	☐
	☐	☐
	☐	☐

Where do you feel it?

Front | *Back*

What about your...?

Mood	1	2	3	4	5	6	7	8	9	10
Energy levels	1	2	3	4	5	6	7	8	9	10
Mental clarity	1	2	3	4	5	6	7	8	9	10

Feeling sick?

☐ Nope!

☐ Yes...

☐ Nausea	☐ Diarrhea	☐ Vomiting	☐ Sore throat
☐ Congestion	☐ Coughing	☐ Chills	☐ Fever

Other symptoms: ______________________________

LET'S EXPLORE SOME MORE

Hours of Sleep	1	2	3	4	5	6	7	8	9	10	+
Sleep Quality	1	2	3	4	5	6	7	8	9	10	

WEATHER

- ☐ Hot ☐ Mild ☐ Cold BM Pressure: ____
- ☐ Dry ☐ Humid ☐ Wet Allergen Levels: ____

STRESS LEVELS

None	Low	Medium	High	Max	@$#%!

FOOD / MEDICATIONS

FOOD / DRINKS

MEDS / SUPPLEMENTS	TIME	DOSE

☐ usual daily medication

EXERCISE / DAILY ACTIVITY

- ☐ Heck yes, I worked out.
- ☐ I managed to exercise a bit.
- ☐ No, I haven't exercised at all.
- ☐ I did some stuff, and that counts.

DETAILS

NOTES / TRIGGERS / IMPROVEMENTS

WRITE ONE THING YOU'RE GRATEFUL FOR

Date: ______________

HOW ARE YOU FEELING TODAY?

					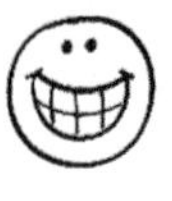	
Like death	Terrible	Not good	Meh	Good	Great!	Amazing!

RATE YOUR PAIN LEVEL

① ② ③ ④ ⑤ ⑥ ⑦ ⑧ ⑨ ⑩

Describe your pain / symptoms	am	pm
	☐	☐
	☐	☐
	☐	☐
	☐	☐
	☐	☐
	☐	☐
	☐	☐
	☐	☐

Where do you feel it?

Front *Back*

What about your…?

Mood	① ② ③ ④ ⑤ ⑥ ⑦ ⑧ ⑨ ⑩
Energy levels	① ② ③ ④ ⑤ ⑥ ⑦ ⑧ ⑨ ⑩
Mental clarity	① ② ③ ④ ⑤ ⑥ ⑦ ⑧ ⑨ ⑩

Feeling sick?

☐ Nope!
☐ Yes…

☐ Nausea	☐ Diarrhea	☐ Vomiting	☐ Sore throat
☐ Congestion	☐ Coughing	☐ Chills	☐ Fever

Other symptoms: ______________________________

LET'S EXPLORE SOME MORE #9

Hours of Sleep	1 2 3 4 5 6 7 8 9 10 +
Sleep Quality	1 2 3 4 5 6 7 8 9 10

WEATHER

☐ Hot ☐ Mild ☐ Cold BM Pressure: ____

☐ Dry ☐ Humid ☐ Wet Allergen Levels: ____

STRESS LEVELS

None	Low	Medium	High	Max	@$#%!

FOOD / MEDICATIONS

FOOD / DRINKS

MEDS / SUPPLEMENTS	TIME	DOSE

☐ usual daily medication

EXERCISE / DAILY ACTIVITY

☐ Heck yes, I worked out.

☐ I managed to exercise a bit.

☐ No, I haven't exercised at all.

☐ I did some stuff, and that counts.

DETAILS

NOTES / TRIGGERS / IMPROVEMENTS

WRITE ONE THING YOU'RE GRATEFUL FOR

Date:______________

HOW ARE YOU FEELING TODAY?

Like death

Terrible

Not good

Meh

Good

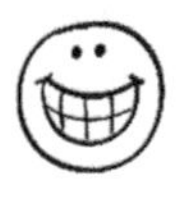
Great!

Amazing!

RATE YOUR PAIN LEVEL

(1) (2) (3) (4) (5) (6) (7) (8) (9) (10)

Describe your pain / symptoms

	am	pm
	☐	☐
	☐	☐
	☐	☐
	☐	☐
	☐	☐
	☐	☐
	☐	☐
	☐	☐

Where do you feel it?

Front

Back

What about your...?

Mood	1	2	3	4	5	6	7	8	9	10
Energy levels	1	2	3	4	5	6	7	8	9	10
Mental clarity	1	2	3	4	5	6	7	8	9	10

Feeling sick?

☐ Nope!

☐ Yes...

☐ Nausea ☐ Diarrhea ☐ Vomiting ☐ Sore throat

☐ Congestion ☐ Coughing ☐ Chills ☐ Fever

Other symptoms: ______________

LET'S EXPLORE SOME MORE

Hours of Sleep	1	2	3	4	5	6	7	8	9	10	+
Sleep Quality	1	2	3	4	5	6	7	8	9	10	

WEATHER

- [ ] Hot
- [ ] Mild
- [ ] Cold
- [ ] Dry
- [ ] Humid
- [ ] Wet

BM Pressure: ______

Allergen Levels: ______

STRESS LEVELS

None	Low	Medium	High	Max	@$#%!

FOOD / MEDICATIONS

FOOD / DRINKS

MEDS / SUPPLEMENTS	TIME	DOSE

- [ ] usual daily medication

EXERCISE / DAILY ACTIVITY

- [ ] Heck yes, I worked out.
- [ ] I managed to exercise a bit.
- [ ] No, I haven't exercised at all.
- [ ] I did some stuff, and that counts.

DETAILS

NOTES / TRIGGERS / IMPROVEMENTS

WRITE ONE THING YOU'RE GRATEFUL FOR

Date: ______________

HOW ARE YOU FEELING TODAY?

Like death	Terrible	Not good	Meh	Good	Great!	Amazing!

RATE YOUR PAIN LEVEL

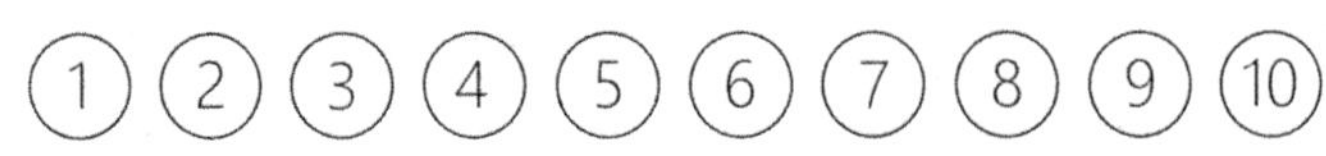

Describe your pain / symptoms	am	pm	Where do you feel it? Front	Back
	☐	☐		
	☐	☐		
	☐	☐		
	☐	☐		
	☐	☐		
	☐	☐		
	☐	☐		
	☐	☐		

What about your...?

Mood	① ② ③ ④ ⑤ ⑥ ⑦ ⑧ ⑨ ⑩
Energy levels	① ② ③ ④ ⑤ ⑥ ⑦ ⑧ ⑨ ⑩
Mental clarity	① ② ③ ④ ⑤ ⑥ ⑦ ⑧ ⑨ ⑩

Feeling sick?

☐ Nope!

☐ Yes...

☐ Nausea	☐ Diarrhea	☐ Vomiting	☐ Sore throat
☐ Congestion	☐ Coughing	☐ Chills	☐ Fever

Other symptoms: ______________________________

LET'S EXPLORE SOME MORE

Hours of Sleep	1	2	3	4	5	6	7	8	9	10	+
Sleep Quality	1	2	3	4	5	6	7	8	9	10	

WEATHER

☐ Hot ☐ Mild ☐ Cold BM Pressure: ____

☐ Dry ☐ Humid ☐ Wet Allergen Levels: ____

STRESS LEVELS

None Low Medium High Max @$#%!

FOOD / MEDICATIONS

FOOD / DRINKS

MEDS / SUPPLEMENTS	TIME	DOSE

☐ usual daily medication

EXERCISE / DAILY ACTIVITY

☐ Heck yes, I worked out.

☐ I managed to exercise a bit.

☐ No, I haven't exercised at all.

☐ I did some stuff, and that counts.

DETAILS

NOTES / TRIGGERS / IMPROVEMENTS

WRITE ONE THING YOU'RE GRATEFUL FOR

Date:______________

HOW ARE YOU FEELING TODAY?

					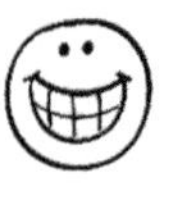	
Like death	Terrible	Not good	Meh	Good	Great!	Amazing!

RATE YOUR PAIN LEVEL

① ② ③ ④ ⑤ ⑥ ⑦ ⑧ ⑨ ⑩

Describe your pain / symptoms	am	pm
	☐	☐
	☐	☐
	☐	☐
	☐	☐
	☐	☐
	☐	☐
	☐	☐
	☐	☐

Where do you feel it?

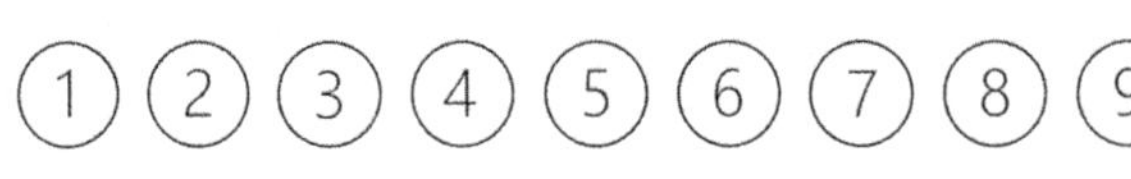

Front *Back*

What about your...?

Mood	① ② ③ ④ ⑤ ⑥ ⑦ ⑧ ⑨ ⑩
Energy levels	① ② ③ ④ ⑤ ⑥ ⑦ ⑧ ⑨ ⑩
Mental clarity	① ② ③ ④ ⑤ ⑥ ⑦ ⑧ ⑨ ⑩

Feeling sick?

☐ Nope!

☐ Yes...

☐ Nausea	☐ Diarrhea	☐ Vomiting	☐ Sore throat
☐ Congestion	☐ Coughing	☐ Chills	☐ Fever

Other symptoms: ______________________

LET'S EXPLORE SOME MORE #12

Hours of Sleep	1 2 3 4 5 6 7 8 9 10 +
Sleep Quality	1 2 3 4 5 6 7 8 9 10

WEATHER

☐ Hot ☐ Mild ☐ Cold BM Pressure: ____

☐ Dry ☐ Humid ☐ Wet Allergen Levels: ____

STRESS LEVELS

None	Low	Medium	High	Max	@$#%!

FOOD / MEDICATIONS

FOOD / DRINKS

MEDS / SUPPLEMENTS	TIME	DOSE

☐ usual daily medication

EXERCISE / DAILY ACTIVITY

☐ Heck yes, I worked out.

☐ I managed to exercise a bit.

☐ No, I haven't exercised at all.

☐ I did some stuff, and that counts.

DETAILS

NOTES / TRIGGERS / IMPROVEMENTS

WRITE ONE THING YOU'RE GRATEFUL FOR

Date:______________

HOW ARE YOU FEELING TODAY?

Like death	Terrible	Not good	Meh	Good	Great!	Amazing!

RATE YOUR PAIN LEVEL

1 2 3 4 5 6 7 8 9 10

Describe your pain / symptoms	am	pm
	☐	☐
	☐	☐
	☐	☐
	☐	☐
	☐	☐
	☐	☐
	☐	☐
	☐	☐

Where do you feel it?

Front *Back*

What about your...?

Mood	1 2 3 4 5 6 7 8 9 10
Energy levels	1 2 3 4 5 6 7 8 9 10
Mental clarity	1 2 3 4 5 6 7 8 9 10

Feeling sick?

☐ Nope!

☐ Yes...

☐ Nausea	☐ Diarrhea	☐ Vomiting	☐ Sore throat
☐ Congestion	☐ Coughing	☐ Chills	☐ Fever

Other symptoms: ____________________

LET'S EXPLORE SOME MORE #13

Hours of Sleep	① ② ③ ④ ⑤ ⑥ ⑦ ⑧ ⑨ ⑩ (+)
Sleep Quality	① ② ③ ④ ⑤ ⑥ ⑦ ⑧ ⑨ ⑩

WEATHER

☐ Hot ☐ Mild ☐ Cold BM Pressure: ____

☐ Dry ☐ Humid ☐ Wet Allergen Levels: ____

STRESS LEVELS

None	Low	Medium	High	Max	@$#%!

FOOD / MEDICATIONS

FOOD / DRINKS

MEDS / SUPPLEMENTS	TIME	DOSE

☐ usual daily medication

EXERCISE / DAILY ACTIVITY

☐ Heck yes, I worked out.

☐ I managed to exercise a bit.

☐ No, I haven't exercised at all.

☐ I did some stuff, and that counts.

DETAILS

NOTES / TRIGGERS / IMPROVEMENTS

WRITE ONE THING YOU'RE GRATEFUL FOR

Date: ______________

HOW ARE YOU FEELING TODAY?

Like death	Terrible	Not good	Meh	Good	Great!	Amazing!

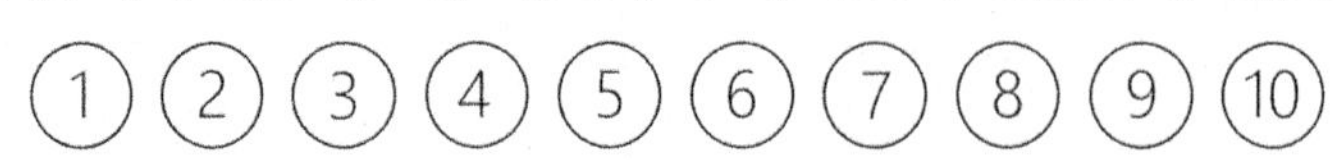

RATE YOUR PAIN LEVEL

① ② ③ ④ ⑤ ⑥ ⑦ ⑧ ⑨ ⑩

Describe your pain / symptoms	am	pm
	☐	☐
	☐	☐
	☐	☐
	☐	☐
	☐	☐
	☐	☐
	☐	☐
	☐	☐

Where do you feel it?

Front *Back*

What about your...?

Mood	1	2	3	4	5	6	7	8	9	10
Energy levels	1	2	3	4	5	6	7	8	9	10
Mental clarity	1	2	3	4	5	6	7	8	9	10

Feeling sick?

☐ Nope!

☐ Yes...

☐ Nausea	☐ Diarrhea	☐ Vomiting	☐ Sore throat
☐ Congestion	☐ Coughing	☐ Chills	☐ Fever

Other symptoms: ______________________________

LET'S EXPLORE SOME MORE

#14

Hours of Sleep	1 2 3 4 5 6 7 8 9 10 +
Sleep Quality	1 2 3 4 5 6 7 8 9 10

WEATHER

- ☐ Hot ☐ Mild ☐ Cold BM Pressure: ____
- ☐ Dry ☐ Humid ☐ Wet Allergen Levels: ____

STRESS LEVELS

None	Low	Medium	High	Max	@$#%!

FOOD / MEDICATIONS

FOOD / DRINKS

MEDS / SUPPLEMENTS	TIME	DOSE

☐ usual daily medication

EXERCISE / DAILY ACTIVITY

- ☐ Heck yes, I worked out.
- ☐ I managed to exercise a bit.
- ☐ No, I haven't exercised at all.
- ☐ I did some stuff, and that counts.

DETAILS

NOTES / TRIGGERS / IMPROVEMENTS

WRITE ONE THING YOU'RE GRATEFUL FOR

Date: _______________

HOW ARE YOU FEELING TODAY?

Like death

Terrible

Not good

Meh

Good

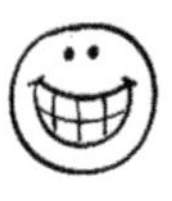
Great!

Amazing!

RATE YOUR PAIN LEVEL

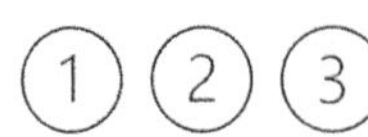 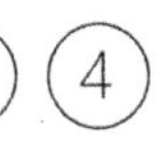 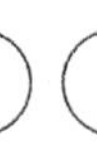 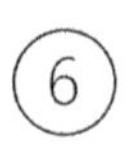 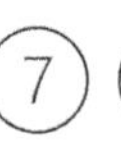 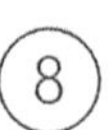 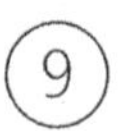 

Describe your pain / symptoms

	am	pm
	☐	☐
	☐	☐
	☐	☐
	☐	☐
	☐	☐
	☐	☐
	☐	☐
	☐	☐

Where do you feel it?

Front *Back*

What about your...?

Mood	① ② ③ ④ ⑤ ⑥ ⑦ ⑧ ⑨ ⑩
Energy levels	① ② ③ ④ ⑤ ⑥ ⑦ ⑧ ⑨ ⑩
Mental clarity	① ② ③ ④ ⑤ ⑥ ⑦ ⑧ ⑨ ⑩

Feeling sick?

☐ Nope!

☐ Yes...

☐ Nausea ☐ Diarrhea ☐ Vomiting ☐ Sore throat

☐ Congestion ☐ Coughing ☐ Chills ☐ Fever

Other symptoms: ______________________

LET'S EXPLORE SOME MORE #15

Hours of Sleep	1	2	3	4	5	6	7	8	9	10	+
Sleep Quality	1	2	3	4	5	6	7	8	9	10	

WEATHER

- ☐ Hot ☐ Mild ☐ Cold BM Pressure: ____
- ☐ Dry ☐ Humid ☐ Wet Allergen Levels: ____

STRESS LEVELS

None	Low	Medium	High	Max	@$#%!

FOOD / MEDICATIONS

FOOD / DRINKS

MEDS / SUPPLEMENTS	TIME	DOSE

☐ usual daily medication

EXERCISE / DAILY ACTIVITY

- ☐ Heck yes, I worked out.
- ☐ I managed to exercise a bit.
- ☐ No, I haven't exercised at all.
- ☐ I did some stuff, and that counts.

DETAILS

NOTES / TRIGGERS / IMPROVEMENTS

WRITE ONE THING YOU'RE GRATEFUL FOR

Date:______________

HOW ARE YOU FEELING TODAY?

Like death | Terrible | Not good | Meh | Good | Great! | Amazing!

RATE YOUR PAIN LEVEL

(1) (2) (3) (4) (5) (6) (7) (8) (9) (10)

Describe your pain / symptoms	am	pm
	☐	☐
	☐	☐
	☐	☐
	☐	☐
	☐	☐
	☐	☐
	☐	☐
	☐	☐

Where do you feel it?

Front *Back*

What about your...?										
Mood	1	2	3	4	5	6	7	8	9	10
Energy levels	1	2	3	4	5	6	7	8	9	10
Mental clarity	1	2	3	4	5	6	7	8	9	10

Feeling sick?

☐ Nope!
☐ Yes...

☐ Nausea ☐ Diarrhea ☐ Vomiting ☐ Sore throat
☐ Congestion ☐ Coughing ☐ Chills ☐ Fever

Other symptoms: ______________________

LET'S EXPLORE SOME MORE #16

Hours of Sleep (1) (2) (3) (4) (5) (6) (7) (8) (9) (10) (+)

Sleep Quality (1) (2) (3) (4) (5) (6) (7) (8) (9) (10)

WEATHER

☐ Hot ☐ Mild ☐ Cold BM Pressure: ____

☐ Dry ☐ Humid ☐ Wet Allergen Levels: ____

STRESS LEVELS

None	Low	Medium	High	Max	@$#%!

FOOD / MEDICATIONS

FOOD / DRINKS

MEDS / SUPPLEMENTS	TIME	DOSE

☐ usual daily medication

EXERCISE / DAILY ACTIVITY

☐ Heck yes, I worked out.

☐ I managed to exercise a bit.

☐ No, I haven't exercised at all.

☐ I did some stuff, and that counts.

DETAILS

NOTES / TRIGGERS / IMPROVEMENTS

WRITE ONE THING YOU'RE GRATEFUL FOR

Date: _______________

HOW ARE YOU FEELING TODAY?

Like death	Terrible	Not good	Meh	Good	Great!	Amazing!

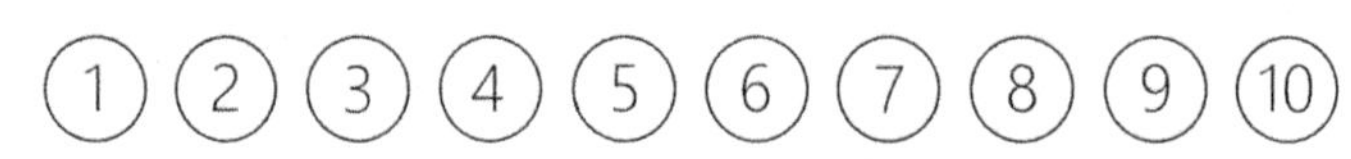

RATE YOUR PAIN LEVEL

(1) (2) (3) (4) (5) (6) (7) (8) (9) (10)

Describe your pain / symptoms

	am	pm
	☐	☐
	☐	☐
	☐	☐
	☐	☐
	☐	☐
	☐	☐
	☐	☐
	☐	☐

Where do you feel it?

Front *Back*

What about your...?

Mood	1	2	3	4	5	6	7	8	9	10
Energy levels	1	2	3	4	5	6	7	8	9	10
Mental clarity	1	2	3	4	5	6	7	8	9	10

Feeling sick?

☐ Nope!

☐ Yes...

☐ Nausea	☐ Diarrhea	☐ Vomiting	☐ Sore throat
☐ Congestion	☐ Coughing	☐ Chills	☐ Fever

Other symptoms: _______________

LET'S EXPLORE SOME MORE #17

Hours of Sleep	① ② ③ ④ ⑤ ⑥ ⑦ ⑧ ⑨ ⑩ ⊕
Sleep Quality	① ② ③ ④ ⑤ ⑥ ⑦ ⑧ ⑨ ⑩

WEATHER

☐ Hot ☐ Mild ☐ Cold BM Pressure: ______

☐ Dry ☐ Humid ☐ Wet Allergen Levels: ______

STRESS LEVELS

None	Low	Medium	High	Max	@$#%!

FOOD / MEDICATIONS

FOOD / DRINKS

MEDS / SUPPLEMENTS	TIME	DOSE

☐ usual daily medication

EXERCISE / DAILY ACTIVITY

☐ Heck yes, I worked out.

☐ I managed to exercise a bit.

☐ No, I haven't exercised at all.

☐ I did some stuff, and that counts.

DETAILS

NOTES / TRIGGERS / IMPROVEMENTS

WRITE ONE THING YOU'RE GRATEFUL FOR

Date: _______________

HOW ARE YOU FEELING TODAY?

Like death	Terrible	Not good	Meh	Good	Great!	Amazing!

RATE YOUR PAIN LEVEL

① ② ③ ④ ⑤ ⑥ ⑦ ⑧ ⑨ ⑩

Describe your pain / symptoms	am	pm
	☐	☐
	☐	☐
	☐	☐
	☐	☐
	☐	☐
	☐	☐
	☐	☐
	☐	☐

Where do you feel it?

Front *Back*

What about your...?

Mood	① ② ③ ④ ⑤ ⑥ ⑦ ⑧ ⑨ ⑩
Energy levels	① ② ③ ④ ⑤ ⑥ ⑦ ⑧ ⑨ ⑩
Mental clarity	① ② ③ ④ ⑤ ⑥ ⑦ ⑧ ⑨ ⑩

Feeling sick?

☐ Nope!

☐ Yes...

☐ Nausea ☐ Diarrhea ☐ Vomiting ☐ Sore throat

☐ Congestion ☐ Coughing ☐ Chills ☐ Fever

Other symptoms: _______________

LET'S EXPLORE SOME MORE #18

Hours of Sleep	1 2 3 4 5 6 7 8 9 10 +
Sleep Quality	1 2 3 4 5 6 7 8 9 10

WEATHER

☐ Hot ☐ Mild ☐ Cold BM Pressure: ____

☐ Dry ☐ Humid ☐ Wet Allergen Levels: ____

STRESS LEVELS

None	Low	Medium	High	Max	@$#%!

FOOD / MEDICATIONS

FOOD / DRINKS

MEDS / SUPPLEMENTS	TIME	DOSE

☐ usual daily medication

EXERCISE / DAILY ACTIVITY

☐ Heck yes, I worked out.

☐ I managed to exercise a bit.

☐ No, I haven't exercised at all.

☐ I did some stuff, and that counts.

DETAILS

NOTES / TRIGGERS / IMPROVEMENTS

WRITE ONE THING YOU'RE GRATEFUL FOR

Date:______________

HOW ARE YOU FEELING TODAY?

Like death

Terrible

Not good

Meh

Good

Great!

Amazing!

RATE YOUR PAIN LEVEL

1 2 3 4 5 6 7 8 9 10

Describe your pain / symptoms	am	pm
	☐	☐
	☐	☐
	☐	☐
	☐	☐
	☐	☐
	☐	☐
	☐	☐
	☐	☐

Where do you feel it?

Front *Back*

What about your...?

Mood	1 2 3 4 5 6 7 8 9 10
Energy levels	1 2 3 4 5 6 7 8 9 10
Mental clarity	1 2 3 4 5 6 7 8 9 10

Feeling sick?

☐ Nope!

☐ Yes...

☐ Nausea	☐ Diarrhea	☐ Vomiting	☐ Sore throat
☐ Congestion	☐ Coughing	☐ Chills	☐ Fever

Other symptoms: ______________________________

LET'S EXPLORE SOME MORE

#19

Hours of Sleep	(1) (2) (3) (4) (5) (6) (7) (8) (9) (10) (+)
Sleep Quality	(1) (2) (3) (4) (5) (6) (7) (8) (9) (10)

WEATHER

- ☐ Hot ☐ Mild ☐ Cold BM Pressure: ____
- ☐ Dry ☐ Humid ☐ Wet Allergen Levels: ____

STRESS LEVELS

None	Low	Medium	High	Max	@$#%!

FOOD / MEDICATIONS

FOOD / DRINKS

MEDS / SUPPLEMENTS	TIME	DOSE

☐ usual daily medication

EXERCISE / DAILY ACTIVITY

- ☐ Heck yes, I worked out.
- ☐ I managed to exercise a bit.
- ☐ No, I haven't exercised at all.
- ☐ I did some stuff, and that counts.

DETAILS

NOTES / TRIGGERS / IMPROVEMENTS

WRITE ONE THING YOU'RE GRATEFUL FOR

Date: ______________

HOW ARE YOU FEELING TODAY?

     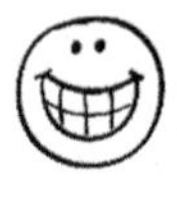 

Like death Terrible Not good Meh Good Great! Amazing!

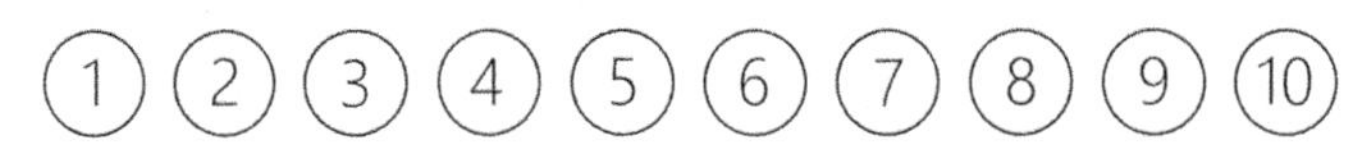

RATE YOUR PAIN LEVEL

① ② ③ ④ ⑤ ⑥ ⑦ ⑧ ⑨ ⑩

Describe your pain / symptoms	am	pm	Where do you feel it? Front	Back
	☐	☐		
	☐	☐		
	☐	☐		
	☐	☐		
	☐	☐		
	☐	☐		
	☐	☐		
	☐	☐		

What about your...?		Feeling sick?
Mood	1 2 3 4 5 6 7 8 9 10	☐ Nope!
Energy levels	1 2 3 4 5 6 7 8 9 10	☐ Yes...
Mental clarity	1 2 3 4 5 6 7 8 9 10	

☐ Nausea ☐ Diarrhea ☐ Vomiting ☐ Sore throat

☐ Congestion ☐ Coughing ☐ Chills ☐ Fever

Other symptoms: ______________________________

LET'S EXPLORE SOME MORE

Hours of Sleep	(1) (2) (3) (4) (5) (6) (7) (8) (9) (10) (+)
Sleep Quality	(1) (2) (3) (4) (5) (6) (7) (8) (9) (10)

WEATHER

☐ Hot	☐ Mild	☐ Cold	BM Pressure: ____
☐ Dry	☐ Humid	☐ Wet	Allergen Levels: ____

STRESS LEVELS

None	Low	Medium	High	Max	@$#%!

FOOD / MEDICATIONS

FOOD / DRINKS

MEDS / SUPPLEMENTS	TIME	DOSE

☐ usual daily medication

EXERCISE / DAILY ACTIVITY

- ☐ Heck yes, I worked out.
- ☐ I managed to exercise a bit.
- ☐ No, I haven't exercised at all.
- ☐ I did some stuff, and that counts.

DETAILS

NOTES / TRIGGERS / IMPROVEMENTS

WRITE ONE THING YOU'RE GRATEFUL FOR

Date: _______________

HOW ARE YOU FEELING TODAY?

Like death · Terrible · Not good · Meh · Good · Great! · Amazing!

RATE YOUR PAIN LEVEL

① ② ③ ④ ⑤ ⑥ ⑦ ⑧ ⑨ ⑩

Describe your pain / symptoms	am	pm	Where do you feel it? Front	Back
	☐	☐		
	☐	☐		
	☐	☐		
	☐	☐		
	☐	☐		
	☐	☐		
	☐	☐		
	☐	☐		

What about your...?		Feeling sick?
Mood	① ② ③ ④ ⑤ ⑥ ⑦ ⑧ ⑨ ⑩	☐ Nope!
Energy levels	① ② ③ ④ ⑤ ⑥ ⑦ ⑧ ⑨ ⑩	☐ Yes...
Mental clarity	① ② ③ ④ ⑤ ⑥ ⑦ ⑧ ⑨ ⑩	

☐ Nausea ☐ Diarrhea ☐ Vomiting ☐ Sore throat
☐ Congestion ☐ Coughing ☐ Chills ☐ Fever

Other symptoms: _______________

LET'S EXPLORE SOME MORE

#21

Hours of Sleep	1	2	3	4	5	6	7	8	9	10	+
Sleep Quality	1	2	3	4	5	6	7	8	9	10	

WEATHER

- ☐ Hot ☐ Mild ☐ Cold BM Pressure: ____
- ☐ Dry ☐ Humid ☐ Wet Allergen Levels: ____

STRESS LEVELS

None	Low	Medium	High	Max	@$#%!

FOOD / MEDICATIONS

FOOD / DRINKS

MEDS / SUPPLEMENTS	TIME	DOSE

☐ usual daily medication

EXERCISE / DAILY ACTIVITY

- ☐ Heck yes, I worked out.
- ☐ I managed to exercise a bit.
- ☐ No, I haven't exercised at all.
- ☐ I did some stuff, and that counts.

DETAILS

NOTES / TRIGGERS / IMPROVEMENTS

WRITE ONE THING YOU'RE GRATEFUL FOR

*Date:*______________

HOW ARE YOU FEELING TODAY?

     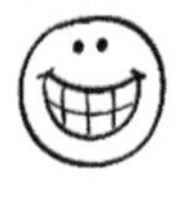 

Like death	Terrible	Not good	Meh	Good	Great!	Amazing!

RATE YOUR PAIN LEVEL

(1) (2) (3) (4) (5) (6) (7) (8) (9) (10)

Describe your pain / symptoms	am	pm	Where do you feel it? Front	Back
	☐	☐		
	☐	☐		
	☐	☐		
	☐	☐		
	☐	☐		
	☐	☐		
	☐	☐		
	☐	☐		

What about your...?

	1	2	3	4	5	6	7	8	9	10
Mood	(1)	(2)	(3)	(4)	(5)	(6)	(7)	(8)	(9)	(10)
Energy levels	(1)	(2)	(3)	(4)	(5)	(6)	(7)	(8)	(9)	(10)
Mental clarity	(1)	(2)	(3)	(4)	(5)	(6)	(7)	(8)	(9)	(10)

Feeling sick?

☐ Nope!

☐ Yes...

☐ Nausea ☐ Diarrhea ☐ Vomiting ☐ Sore throat

☐ Congestion ☐ Coughing ☐ Chills ☐ Fever

Other symptoms: ______________________

LET'S EXPLORE SOME MORE #22

Hours of Sleep	1	2	3	4	5	6	7	8	9	10	+
Sleep Quality	1	2	3	4	5	6	7	8	9	10	

WEATHER

- ☐ Hot ☐ Mild ☐ Cold BM Pressure: ______
- ☐ Dry ☐ Humid ☐ Wet Allergen Levels: ______

STRESS LEVELS

None	Low	Medium	High	Max	@$#%!

FOOD / MEDICATIONS

FOOD / DRINKS

MEDS / SUPPLEMENTS	TIME	DOSE

☐ usual daily medication

EXERCISE / DAILY ACTIVITY

- ☐ Heck yes, I worked out.
- ☐ I managed to exercise a bit.
- ☐ No, I haven't exercised at all.
- ☐ I did some stuff, and that counts.

DETAILS

NOTES / TRIGGERS / IMPROVEMENTS

WRITE ONE THING YOU'RE GRATEFUL FOR

Date: ______________

HOW ARE YOU FEELING TODAY?

					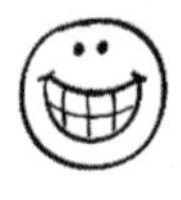	
Like death	Terrible	Not good	Meh	Good	Great!	Amazing!

RATE YOUR PAIN LEVEL

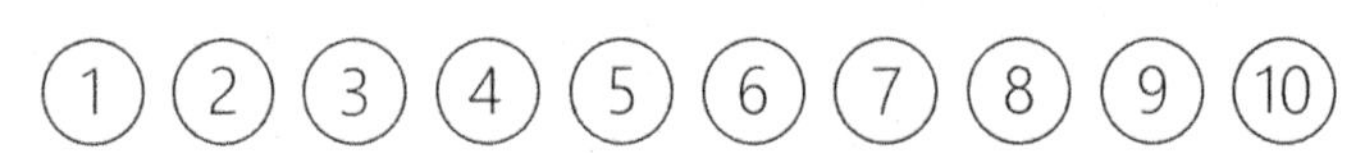

Describe your pain / symptoms	am	pm	Where do you feel it? Front	Back
	☐	☐		
	☐	☐		
	☐	☐		
	☐	☐		
	☐	☐		
	☐	☐		
	☐	☐		
	☐	☐		

What about your...?		Feeling sick?
Mood	① ② ③ ④ ⑤ ⑥ ⑦ ⑧ ⑨ ⑩	☐ Nope!
Energy levels	① ② ③ ④ ⑤ ⑥ ⑦ ⑧ ⑨ ⑩	☐ Yes...
Mental clarity	① ② ③ ④ ⑤ ⑥ ⑦ ⑧ ⑨ ⑩	

☐ Nausea	☐ Diarrhea	☐ Vomiting	☐ Sore throat
☐ Congestion	☐ Coughing	☐ Chills	☐ Fever

Other symptoms: ______________________________

LET'S EXPLORE SOME MORE #23

Hours of Sleep	1	2	3	4	5	6	7	8	9	10	+
Sleep Quality	1	2	3	4	5	6	7	8	9	10	

WEATHER

☐ Hot ☐ Mild ☐ Cold BM Pressure: ____

☐ Dry ☐ Humid ☐ Wet Allergen Levels: ____

STRESS LEVELS

None	Low	Medium	High	Max	@$#%!

FOOD / MEDICATIONS

FOOD / DRINKS

MEDS / SUPPLEMENTS	TIME	DOSE

☐ usual daily medication

EXERCISE / DAILY ACTIVITY

☐ Heck yes, I worked out.

☐ I managed to exercise a bit.

☐ No, I haven't exercised at all.

☐ I did some stuff, and that counts.

DETAILS

NOTES / TRIGGERS / IMPROVEMENTS

WRITE ONE THING YOU'RE GRATEFUL FOR

Date: ______________

HOW ARE YOU FEELING TODAY?

Like death	Terrible	Not good	Meh	Good	Great!	Amazing!

RATE YOUR PAIN LEVEL

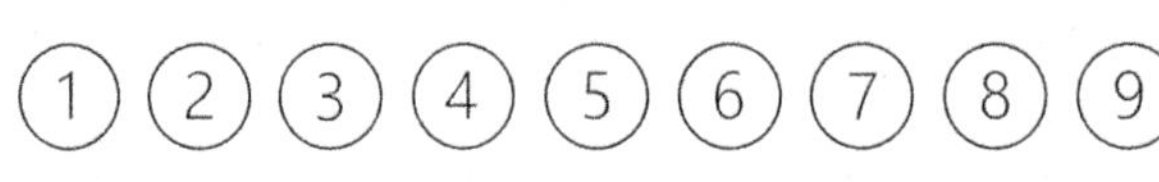

Describe your pain / symptoms

	am	pm
	☐	☐
	☐	☐
	☐	☐
	☐	☐
	☐	☐
	☐	☐
	☐	☐
	☐	☐

Where do you feel it?

Front *Back*

What about your...?

Mood	1	2	3	4	5	6	7	8	9	10
Energy levels	1	2	3	4	5	6	7	8	9	10
Mental clarity	1	2	3	4	5	6	7	8	9	10

Feeling sick?

☐ Nope!

☐ Yes...

☐ Nausea ☐ Diarrhea ☐ Vomiting ☐ Sore throat

☐ Congestion ☐ Coughing ☐ Chills ☐ Fever

Other symptoms: ______________________________

LET'S EXPLORE SOME MORE #24

Hours of Sleep	1	2	3	4	5	6	7	8	9	10	+
Sleep Quality	1	2	3	4	5	6	7	8	9	10	

WEATHER

- [ ] Hot
- [ ] Mild
- [ ] Cold

BM Pressure: ____

- [ ] Dry
- [ ] Humid
- [ ] Wet

Allergen Levels: ____

STRESS LEVELS

None	Low	Medium	High	Max	@$#%!

FOOD / MEDICATIONS

FOOD / DRINKS

MEDS / SUPPLEMENTS	TIME	DOSE

- [ ] usual daily medication

EXERCISE / DAILY ACTIVITY

- [ ] Heck yes, I worked out.
- [ ] I managed to exercise a bit.
- [ ] No, I haven't exercised at all.
- [ ] I did some stuff, and that counts.

DETAILS

NOTES / TRIGGERS / IMPROVEMENTS

WRITE ONE THING YOU'RE GRATEFUL FOR

Date:______________

HOW ARE YOU FEELING TODAY?

Like death

Terrible

Not good

Meh

Good

Great!

Amazing!

RATE YOUR PAIN LEVEL

(1) (2) (3) (4) (5) (6) (7) (8) (9) (10)

Describe your pain / symptoms	am	pm	Where do you feel it? Front	Back
	☐	☐		
	☐	☐		
	☐	☐		
	☐	☐		
	☐	☐		
	☐	☐		
	☐	☐		
	☐	☐		

What about your...?		Feeling sick?
Mood	(1) (2) (3) (4) (5) (6) (7) (8) (9) (10)	☐ Nope!
Energy levels	(1) (2) (3) (4) (5) (6) (7) (8) (9) (10)	☐ Yes...
Mental clarity	(1) (2) (3) (4) (5) (6) (7) (8) (9) (10)	

☐ Nausea	☐ Diarrhea	☐ Vomiting	☐ Sore throat
☐ Congestion	☐ Coughing	☐ Chills	☐ Fever

Other symptoms: ______________________________

LET'S EXPLORE SOME MORE

#25

Hours of Sleep	1 2 3 4 5 6 7 8 9 10 +
Sleep Quality	1 2 3 4 5 6 7 8 9 10

WEATHER

☐ Hot ☐ Mild ☐ Cold BM Pressure: ____

☐ Dry ☐ Humid ☐ Wet Allergen Levels: ____

STRESS LEVELS

None	Low	Medium	High	Max	@$#%!

FOOD / MEDICATIONS

FOOD / DRINKS

MEDS / SUPPLEMENTS	TIME	DOSE

☐ usual daily medication

EXERCISE / DAILY ACTIVITY

☐ Heck yes, I worked out.

☐ I managed to exercise a bit.

☐ No, I haven't exercised at all.

☐ I did some stuff, and that counts.

DETAILS

NOTES / TRIGGERS / IMPROVEMENTS

WRITE ONE THING YOU'RE GRATEFUL FOR

Date: ______________

HOW ARE YOU FEELING TODAY?

Like death	Terrible	Not good	Meh	Good	Great!	Amazing!

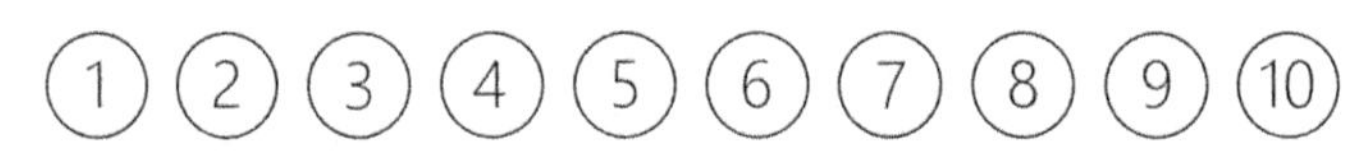

RATE YOUR PAIN LEVEL

① ② ③ ④ ⑤ ⑥ ⑦ ⑧ ⑨ ⑩

Describe your pain / symptoms	am	pm
	☐	☐
	☐	☐
	☐	☐
	☐	☐
	☐	☐
	☐	☐
	☐	☐
	☐	☐

Where do you feel it?

Front *Back*

What about your...?

Mood	① ② ③ ④ ⑤ ⑥ ⑦ ⑧ ⑨ ⑩
Energy levels	① ② ③ ④ ⑤ ⑥ ⑦ ⑧ ⑨ ⑩
Mental clarity	① ② ③ ④ ⑤ ⑥ ⑦ ⑧ ⑨ ⑩

Feeling sick?

☐ Nope!
☐ Yes...

☐ Nausea	☐ Diarrhea	☐ Vomiting	☐ Sore throat
☐ Congestion	☐ Coughing	☐ Chills	☐ Fever

Other symptoms: ______________________

LET'S EXPLORE SOME MORE

Hours of Sleep	1	2	3	4	5	6	7	8	9	10	+
Sleep Quality	1	2	3	4	5	6	7	8	9	10	

WEATHER

- ☐ Hot ☐ Mild ☐ Cold BM Pressure: ______
- ☐ Dry ☐ Humid ☐ Wet Allergen Levels: ______

STRESS LEVELS

None	Low	Medium	High	Max	@$#%!

FOOD / MEDICATIONS

FOOD / DRINKS

MEDS / SUPPLEMENTS	TIME	DOSE

☐ usual daily medication

EXERCISE / DAILY ACTIVITY

- ☐ Heck yes, I worked out.
- ☐ I managed to exercise a bit.
- ☐ No, I haven't exercised at all.
- ☐ I did some stuff, and that counts.

DETAILS

NOTES / TRIGGERS / IMPROVEMENTS

WRITE ONE THING YOU'RE GRATEFUL FOR

Date: ______________

HOW ARE YOU FEELING TODAY?

Like death	Terrible	Not good	Meh	Good	Great!	Amazing!

RATE YOUR PAIN LEVEL

(1) (2) (3) (4) (5) (6) (7) (8) (9) (10)

Describe your pain / symptoms	am	pm	Where do you feel it?	
			Front	*Back*
	☐	☐		
	☐	☐		
	☐	☐		
	☐	☐		
	☐	☐		
	☐	☐		
	☐	☐		
	☐	☐		

What about your...?		Feeling sick?
Mood	(1) (2) (3) (4) (5) (6) (7) (8) (9) (10)	☐ Nope!
Energy levels	(1) (2) (3) (4) (5) (6) (7) (8) (9) (10)	☐ Yes...
Mental clarity	(1) (2) (3) (4) (5) (6) (7) (8) (9) (10)	

☐ Nausea	☐ Diarrhea	☐ Vomiting	☐ Sore throat
☐ Congestion	☐ Coughing	☐ Chills	☐ Fever

Other symptoms: ______________________________

LET'S EXPLORE SOME MORE #27

Hours of Sleep (1) (2) (3) (4) (5) (6) (7) (8) (9) (10) (+)

Sleep Quality (1) (2) (3) (4) (5) (6) (7) (8) (9) (10)

WEATHER

- [ ] Hot - [ ] Mild - [ ] Cold BM Pressure: ____
- [ ] Dry - [ ] Humid - [ ] Wet Allergen Levels: ____

STRESS LEVELS

None Low Medium High Max @$#%!

FOOD / MEDICATIONS

FOOD / DRINKS

MEDS / SUPPLEMENTS	TIME	DOSE

- [ ] usual daily medication

EXERCISE / DAILY ACTIVITY

- [ ] Heck yes, I worked out.
- [ ] I managed to exercise a bit.
- [ ] No, I haven't exercised at all.
- [ ] I did some stuff, and that counts.

DETAILS

NOTES / TRIGGERS / IMPROVEMENTS

WRITE ONE THING YOU'RE GRATEFUL FOR

Date:______________

HOW ARE YOU FEELING TODAY?

     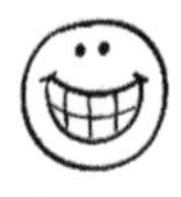 

Like death | Terrible | Not good | Meh | Good | Great! | Amazing!

RATE YOUR PAIN LEVEL

① ② ③ ④ ⑤ ⑥ ⑦ ⑧ ⑨ ⑩

Describe your pain / symptoms	am	pm
	☐	☐
	☐	☐
	☐	☐
	☐	☐
	☐	☐
	☐	☐
	☐	☐
	☐	☐

Where do you feel it?

Front | *Back*

What about your...?

Mood	1 2 3 4 5 6 7 8 9 10
Energy levels	1 2 3 4 5 6 7 8 9 10
Mental clarity	1 2 3 4 5 6 7 8 9 10

Feeling sick?

☐ Nope!
☐ Yes...

☐ Nausea ☐ Diarrhea ☐ Vomiting ☐ Sore throat
☐ Congestion ☐ Coughing ☐ Chills ☐ Fever

Other symptoms: ______________________

LET'S EXPLORE SOME MORE

Hours of Sleep	1	2	3	4	5	6	7	8	9	10	+
Sleep Quality	1	2	3	4	5	6	7	8	9	10	

WEATHER

- ☐ Hot ☐ Mild ☐ Cold BM Pressure: ____
- ☐ Dry ☐ Humid ☐ Wet Allergen Levels: ____

STRESS LEVELS

None	Low	Medium	High	Max	@$#%!

FOOD / MEDICATIONS

FOOD / DRINKS

MEDS / SUPPLEMENTS	TIME	DOSE

☐ usual daily medication

EXERCISE / DAILY ACTIVITY

- ☐ Heck yes, I worked out.
- ☐ I managed to exercise a bit.
- ☐ No, I haven't exercised at all.
- ☐ I did some stuff, and that counts.

DETAILS

NOTES / TRIGGERS / IMPROVEMENTS

WRITE ONE THING YOU'RE GRATEFUL FOR

Date: ______________

HOW ARE YOU FEELING TODAY?

Like death	Terrible	Not good	Meh	Good	Great!	Amazing!

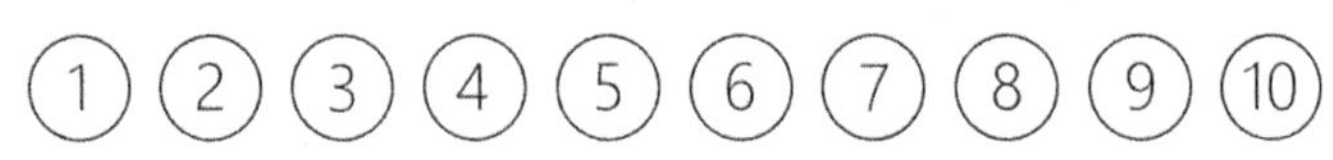

RATE YOUR PAIN LEVEL

① ② ③ ④ ⑤ ⑥ ⑦ ⑧ ⑨ ⑩

Describe your pain / symptoms	am	pm
	☐	☐
	☐	☐
	☐	☐
	☐	☐
	☐	☐
	☐	☐
	☐	☐
	☐	☐

Where do you feel it?

Front *Back*

What about your...?

Mood	1	2	3	4	5	6	7	8	9	10
Energy levels	1	2	3	4	5	6	7	8	9	10
Mental clarity	1	2	3	4	5	6	7	8	9	10

Feeling sick?

☐ Nope!
☐ Yes...

☐ Nausea ☐ Diarrhea ☐ Vomiting ☐ Sore throat
☐ Congestion ☐ Coughing ☐ Chills ☐ Fever

Other symptoms: ______________

LET'S EXPLORE SOME MORE #29

Hours of Sleep	1 2 3 4 5 6 7 8 9 10 +
Sleep Quality	1 2 3 4 5 6 7 8 9 10

WEATHER

- [ ] Hot
- [ ] Mild
- [ ] Cold
- [ ] Dry
- [ ] Humid
- [ ] Wet

BM Pressure: ______

Allergen Levels: ______

STRESS LEVELS

None | Low | Medium | High | Max | @$#%!

FOOD / MEDICATIONS

FOOD / DRINKS

MEDS / SUPPLEMENTS	TIME	DOSE

- [ ] usual daily medication

EXERCISE / DAILY ACTIVITY

- [ ] Heck yes, I worked out.
- [ ] I managed to exercise a bit.
- [ ] No, I haven't exercised at all.
- [ ] I did some stuff, and that counts.

DETAILS

NOTES / TRIGGERS / IMPROVEMENTS

WRITE ONE THING YOU'RE GRATEFUL FOR

Date:______________

HOW ARE YOU FEELING TODAY?

Like death	Terrible	Not good	Meh	Good	Great!	Amazing!

RATE YOUR PAIN LEVEL

① ② ③ ④ ⑤ ⑥ ⑦ ⑧ ⑨ ⑩

Describe your pain / symptoms	am	pm
	☐	☐
	☐	☐
	☐	☐
	☐	☐
	☐	☐
	☐	☐
	☐	☐
	☐	☐

Where do you feel it?

Front *Back*

What about your...?

Mood	1	2	3	4	5	6	7	8	9	10
Energy levels	1	2	3	4	5	6	7	8	9	10
Mental clarity	1	2	3	4	5	6	7	8	9	10

Feeling sick?

☐ Nope!
☐ Yes...

☐ Nausea	☐ Diarrhea	☐ Vomiting	☐ Sore throat
☐ Congestion	☐ Coughing	☐ Chills	☐ Fever

Other symptoms: ____________________

LET'S EXPLORE SOME MORE #30

Hours of Sleep	① ② ③ ④ ⑤ ⑥ ⑦ ⑧ ⑨ ⑩ ⊕
Sleep Quality	① ② ③ ④ ⑤ ⑥ ⑦ ⑧ ⑨ ⑩

WEATHER

☐ Hot ☐ Mild ☐ Cold BM Pressure: ____

☐ Dry ☐ Humid ☐ Wet Allergen Levels: ____

STRESS LEVELS

None	Low	Medium	High	Max	@$#%!

FOOD / MEDICATIONS

FOOD / DRINKS

MEDS / SUPPLEMENTS	TIME	DOSE

☐ usual daily medication

EXERCISE / DAILY ACTIVITY

☐ Heck yes, I worked out.

☐ I managed to exercise a bit.

☐ No, I haven't exercised at all.

☐ I did some stuff, and that counts.

DETAILS

NOTES / TRIGGERS / IMPROVEMENTS

WRITE ONE THING YOU'RE GRATEFUL FOR

Date: ______________

HOW ARE YOU FEELING TODAY?

Like death

Terrible

Not good

Meh

Good

Great!

Amazing!

RATE YOUR PAIN LEVEL

① ② ③ ④ ⑤ ⑥ ⑦ ⑧ ⑨ ⑩

Describe your pain / symptoms	am	pm
	☐	☐
	☐	☐
	☐	☐
	☐	☐
	☐	☐
	☐	☐
	☐	☐
	☐	☐

Where do you feel it?

Front *Back*

What about your...?

Mood	① ② ③ ④ ⑤ ⑥ ⑦ ⑧ ⑨ ⑩
Energy levels	① ② ③ ④ ⑤ ⑥ ⑦ ⑧ ⑨ ⑩
Mental clarity	① ② ③ ④ ⑤ ⑥ ⑦ ⑧ ⑨ ⑩

Feeling sick?

☐ Nope!
☐ Yes...

☐ Nausea ☐ Diarrhea ☐ Vomiting ☐ Sore throat
☐ Congestion ☐ Coughing ☐ Chills ☐ Fever

Other symptoms: ______________________________

LET'S EXPLORE SOME MORE

Hours of Sleep	1 2 3 4 5 6 7 8 9 10 +
Sleep Quality	1 2 3 4 5 6 7 8 9 10

WEATHER

- [ ] Hot
- [ ] Mild
- [ ] Cold
- [ ] Dry
- [ ] Humid
- [ ] Wet

BM Pressure: ______

Allergen Levels: ______

STRESS LEVELS

None	Low	Medium	High	Max	@$#%!

FOOD / MEDICATIONS

FOOD / DRINKS

MEDS / SUPPLEMENTS	TIME	DOSE

- [ ] usual daily medication

EXERCISE / DAILY ACTIVITY

- [ ] Heck yes, I worked out.
- [ ] I managed to exercise a bit.
- [ ] No, I haven't exercised at all.
- [ ] I did some stuff, and that counts.

DETAILS

NOTES / TRIGGERS / IMPROVEMENTS

WRITE ONE THING YOU'RE GRATEFUL FOR

Date: ______________

HOW ARE YOU FEELING TODAY?

Like death	Terrible	Not good	Meh	Good	Great!	Amazing!

RATE YOUR PAIN LEVEL

① ② ③ ④ ⑤ ⑥ ⑦ ⑧ ⑨ ⑩

Describe your pain / symptoms	am	pm	Where do you feel it? Front	Back
	☐	☐		
	☐	☐		
	☐	☐		
	☐	☐		
	☐	☐		
	☐	☐		
	☐	☐		
	☐	☐		

What about your...?

Mood	1	2	3	4	5	6	7	8	9	10
Energy levels	1	2	3	4	5	6	7	8	9	10
Mental clarity	1	2	3	4	5	6	7	8	9	10

Feeling sick?

☐ Nope!
☐ Yes...

☐ Nausea ☐ Diarrhea ☐ Vomiting ☐ Sore throat
☐ Congestion ☐ Coughing ☐ Chills ☐ Fever

Other symptoms: ______________________________

LET'S EXPLORE SOME MORE #32

Hours of Sleep	1	2	3	4	5	6	7	8	9	10	+
Sleep Quality	1	2	3	4	5	6	7	8	9	10	

WEATHER

☐ Hot ☐ Mild ☐ Cold BM Pressure: ____

☐ Dry ☐ Humid ☐ Wet Allergen Levels: ____

STRESS LEVELS

None	Low	Medium	High	Max	@$#%!

FOOD / MEDICATIONS

FOOD / DRINKS

MEDS / SUPPLEMENTS	TIME	DOSE

☐ usual daily medication

EXERCISE / DAILY ACTIVITY

☐ Heck yes, I worked out.

☐ I managed to exercise a bit.

☐ No, I haven't exercised at all.

☐ I did some stuff, and that counts.

DETAILS

NOTES / TRIGGERS / IMPROVEMENTS

WRITE ONE THING YOU'RE GRATEFUL FOR

Date:______________

HOW ARE YOU FEELING TODAY?

     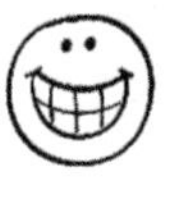 

Like death | Terrible | Not good | Meh | Good | Great! | Amazing!

RATE YOUR PAIN LEVEL

① ② ③ ④ ⑤ ⑥ ⑦ ⑧ ⑨ ⑩

Describe your pain / symptoms	am	pm
	☐	☐
	☐	☐
	☐	☐
	☐	☐
	☐	☐
	☐	☐
	☐	☐
	☐	☐

Where do you feel it?

Front | *Back*

What about your...?

Mood	① ② ③ ④ ⑤ ⑥ ⑦ ⑧ ⑨ ⑩
Energy levels	① ② ③ ④ ⑤ ⑥ ⑦ ⑧ ⑨ ⑩
Mental clarity	① ② ③ ④ ⑤ ⑥ ⑦ ⑧ ⑨ ⑩

Feeling sick?

☐ Nope!
☐ Yes...

☐ Nausea ☐ Diarrhea ☐ Vomiting ☐ Sore throat
☐ Congestion ☐ Coughing ☐ Chills ☐ Fever

Other symptoms: ____________________

LET'S EXPLORE SOME MORE

Hours of Sleep	1	2	3	4	5	6	7	8	9	10	+
Sleep Quality	1	2	3	4	5	6	7	8	9	10	

WEATHER

- ☐ Hot ☐ Mild ☐ Cold BM Pressure: ____
- ☐ Dry ☐ Humid ☐ Wet Allergen Levels: ____

STRESS LEVELS

None	Low	Medium	High	Max	@$#%!

FOOD / MEDICATIONS

FOOD / DRINKS

MEDS / SUPPLEMENTS	TIME	DOSE

☐ usual daily medication

EXERCISE / DAILY ACTIVITY

- ☐ Heck yes, I worked out.
- ☐ I managed to exercise a bit.
- ☐ No, I haven't exercised at all.
- ☐ I did some stuff, and that counts.

DETAILS

NOTES / TRIGGERS / IMPROVEMENTS

WRITE ONE THING YOU'RE GRATEFUL FOR

Date:______________

HOW ARE YOU FEELING TODAY?

 Like death
 Terrible
 Not good
 Meh
 Good
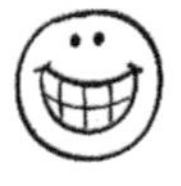 Great!
 Amazing!

RATE YOUR PAIN LEVEL

(1) (2) (3) (4) (5) (6) (7) (8) (9) (10)

Describe your pain / symptoms	am	pm	Where do you feel it?	
	am	pm	*Front*	*Back*
	☐	☐		
	☐	☐		
	☐	☐		
	☐	☐		
	☐	☐		
	☐	☐		
	☐	☐		
	☐	☐		

What about your...?		Feeling sick?
Mood	(1) (2) (3) (4) (5) (6) (7) (8) (9) (10)	☐ Nope!
Energy levels	(1) (2) (3) (4) (5) (6) (7) (8) (9) (10)	☐ Yes...
Mental clarity	(1) (2) (3) (4) (5) (6) (7) (8) (9) (10)	

☐ Nausea ☐ Diarrhea ☐ Vomiting ☐ Sore throat
☐ Congestion ☐ Coughing ☐ Chills ☐ Fever

Other symptoms: ______________________

LET'S EXPLORE SOME MORE #34

Hours of Sleep	1	2	3	4	5	6	7	8	9	10	+
Sleep Quality	1	2	3	4	5	6	7	8	9	10	

WEATHER

- ☐ Hot ☐ Mild ☐ Cold BM Pressure: ______
- ☐ Dry ☐ Humid ☐ Wet Allergen Levels: ______

STRESS LEVELS

None	Low	Medium	High	Max	@$#%!

FOOD / MEDICATIONS

FOOD / DRINKS

MEDS / SUPPLEMENTS	TIME	DOSE

☐ usual daily medication

EXERCISE / DAILY ACTIVITY

- ☐ Heck yes, I worked out.
- ☐ I managed to exercise a bit.
- ☐ No, I haven't exercised at all.
- ☐ I did some stuff, and that counts.

DETAILS

NOTES / TRIGGERS / IMPROVEMENTS

WRITE ONE THING YOU'RE GRATEFUL FOR

Date:______________

HOW ARE YOU FEELING TODAY?

 Like death
 Terrible
 Not good
 Meh
 Good
 Great!
 Amazing!

RATE YOUR PAIN LEVEL

① ② ③ ④ ⑤ ⑥ ⑦ ⑧ ⑨ ⑩

Describe your pain / symptoms	am	pm
	☐	☐
	☐	☐
	☐	☐
	☐	☐
	☐	☐
	☐	☐
	☐	☐
	☐	☐

Where do you feel it?

Front *Back*

What about your...?

Mood	1	2	3	4	5	6	7	8	9	10
Energy levels	1	2	3	4	5	6	7	8	9	10
Mental clarity	1	2	3	4	5	6	7	8	9	10

Feeling sick?

☐ Nope!
☐ Yes...

☐ Nausea ☐ Diarrhea ☐ Vomiting ☐ Sore throat
☐ Congestion ☐ Coughing ☐ Chills ☐ Fever

Other symptoms: ______________________

LET'S EXPLORE SOME MORE

Hours of Sleep	1	2	3	4	5	6	7	8	9	10	+
Sleep Quality	1	2	3	4	5	6	7	8	9	10	

WEATHER

- ☐ Hot ☐ Mild ☐ Cold BM Pressure: ____
- ☐ Dry ☐ Humid ☐ Wet Allergen Levels: ____

STRESS LEVELS

None	Low	Medium	High	Max	@$#%!

FOOD / MEDICATIONS

FOOD / DRINKS

MEDS / SUPPLEMENTS	TIME	DOSE

☐ usual daily medication

EXERCISE / DAILY ACTIVITY

- ☐ Heck yes, I worked out.
- ☐ I managed to exercise a bit.
- ☐ No, I haven't exercised at all.
- ☐ I did some stuff, and that counts.

DETAILS

NOTES / TRIGGERS / IMPROVEMENTS

WRITE ONE THING YOU'RE GRATEFUL FOR

Date: ______________

HOW ARE YOU FEELING TODAY?

Like death

Terrible

Not good

Meh

Good

Great!

Amazing!

RATE YOUR PAIN LEVEL

1 2 3 4 5 6 7 8 9 10

Describe your pain / symptoms	am	pm
	☐	☐
	☐	☐
	☐	☐
	☐	☐
	☐	☐
	☐	☐
	☐	☐
	☐	☐

Where do you feel it?

Front *Back*

What about your...?

Mood	1 2 3 4 5 6 7 8 9 10
Energy levels	1 2 3 4 5 6 7 8 9 10
Mental clarity	1 2 3 4 5 6 7 8 9 10

Feeling sick?

☐ Nope!
☐ Yes...

☐ Nausea	☐ Diarrhea	☐ Vomiting	☐ Sore throat
☐ Congestion	☐ Coughing	☐ Chills	☐ Fever

Other symptoms: ______________________________

LET'S EXPLORE SOME MORE

#36

Hours of Sleep	1	2	3	4	5	6	7	8	9	10	+
Sleep Quality	1	2	3	4	5	6	7	8	9	10	

WEATHER

☐ Hot ☐ Mild ☐ Cold BM Pressure: ____

☐ Dry ☐ Humid ☐ Wet Allergen Levels: ____

STRESS LEVELS

None	Low	Medium	High	Max	@$#%!

FOOD / MEDICATIONS

FOOD / DRINKS

MEDS / SUPPLEMENTS	TIME	DOSE

☐ usual daily medication

EXERCISE / DAILY ACTIVITY

☐ Heck yes, I worked out.

☐ I managed to exercise a bit.

☐ No, I haven't exercised at all.

☐ I did some stuff, and that counts.

DETAILS

NOTES / TRIGGERS / IMPROVEMENTS

WRITE ONE THING YOU'RE GRATEFUL FOR

Date: _____________

HOW ARE YOU FEELING TODAY?

     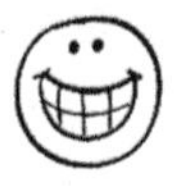 

Like death	Terrible	Not good	Meh	Good	Great!	Amazing!

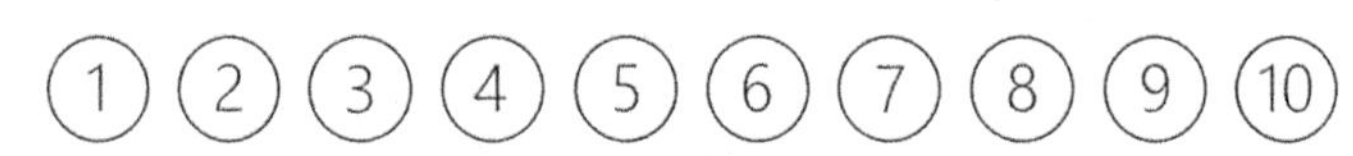

RATE YOUR PAIN LEVEL

① ② ③ ④ ⑤ ⑥ ⑦ ⑧ ⑨ ⑩

Describe your pain / symptoms	am	pm
	☐	☐
	☐	☐
	☐	☐
	☐	☐
	☐	☐
	☐	☐
	☐	☐
	☐	☐

Where do you feel it?

Front *Back*

What about your...?

Mood	1	2	3	4	5	6	7	8	9	10
Energy levels	1	2	3	4	5	6	7	8	9	10
Mental clarity	1	2	3	4	5	6	7	8	9	10

Feeling sick?

☐ Nope!
☐ Yes...

☐ Nausea ☐ Diarrhea ☐ Vomiting ☐ Sore throat
☐ Congestion ☐ Coughing ☐ Chills ☐ Fever

Other symptoms: ______________________

LET'S EXPLORE SOME MORE #37

Hours of Sleep	1	2	3	4	5	6	7	8	9	10	+
Sleep Quality	1	2	3	4	5	6	7	8	9	10	

WEATHER

- [ ] Hot
- [ ] Mild
- [ ] Cold
- [ ] Dry
- [ ] Humid
- [ ] Wet

BM Pressure: ____

Allergen Levels: ____

STRESS LEVELS

None	Low	Medium	High	Max	@$#%!

FOOD / MEDICATIONS

FOOD / DRINKS

MEDS / SUPPLEMENTS	TIME	DOSE

- [ ] usual daily medication

EXERCISE / DAILY ACTIVITY

- [ ] Heck yes, I worked out.
- [ ] I managed to exercise a bit.
- [ ] No, I haven't exercised at all.
- [ ] I did some stuff, and that counts.

DETAILS

NOTES / TRIGGERS / IMPROVEMENTS

WRITE ONE THING YOU'RE GRATEFUL FOR

Date:_____________

HOW ARE YOU FEELING TODAY?

Like death	Terrible	Not good	Meh	Good	Great!	Amazing!

RATE YOUR PAIN LEVEL

① ② ③ ④ ⑤ ⑥ ⑦ ⑧ ⑨ ⑩

Describe your pain / symptoms	am	pm
	☐	☐
	☐	☐
	☐	☐
	☐	☐
	☐	☐
	☐	☐
	☐	☐
	☐	☐

Where do you feel it?

Front *Back*

What about your...?

Mood	① ② ③ ④ ⑤ ⑥ ⑦ ⑧ ⑨ ⑩
Energy levels	① ② ③ ④ ⑤ ⑥ ⑦ ⑧ ⑨ ⑩
Mental clarity	① ② ③ ④ ⑤ ⑥ ⑦ ⑧ ⑨ ⑩

Feeling sick?

☐ Nope!

☐ Yes...

☐ Nausea ☐ Diarrhea ☐ Vomiting ☐ Sore throat

☐ Congestion ☐ Coughing ☐ Chills ☐ Fever

Other symptoms: ____________________

LET'S EXPLORE SOME MORE #38

Hours of Sleep	1	2	3	4	5	6	7	8	9	10	+
Sleep Quality	1	2	3	4	5	6	7	8	9	10	

WEATHER

- ☐ Hot ☐ Mild ☐ Cold BM Pressure: ____
- ☐ Dry ☐ Humid ☐ Wet Allergen Levels: ____

STRESS LEVELS

None	Low	Medium	High	Max	@$#%!

FOOD / MEDICATIONS

FOOD / DRINKS

MEDS / SUPPLEMENTS	TIME	DOSE

☐ usual daily medication

EXERCISE / DAILY ACTIVITY

- ☐ Heck yes, I worked out.
- ☐ I managed to exercise a bit.
- ☐ No, I haven't exercised at all.
- ☐ I did some stuff, and that counts.

DETAILS

NOTES / TRIGGERS / IMPROVEMENTS

WRITE ONE THING YOU'RE GRATEFUL FOR

Date: ______________

HOW ARE YOU FEELING TODAY?

Like death	Terrible	Not good	Meh	Good	Great!	Amazing!

RATE YOUR PAIN LEVEL

(1) (2) (3) (4) (5) (6) (7) (8) (9) (10)

Describe your pain / symptoms	am	pm
	☐	☐
	☐	☐
	☐	☐
	☐	☐
	☐	☐
	☐	☐
	☐	☐
	☐	☐

Where do you feel it?

Front *Back*

What about your...?

Mood	1	2	3	4	5	6	7	8	9	10
Energy levels	1	2	3	4	5	6	7	8	9	10
Mental clarity	1	2	3	4	5	6	7	8	9	10

Feeling sick?

☐ Nope!

☐ Yes...

☐ Nausea ☐ Diarrhea ☐ Vomiting ☐ Sore throat

☐ Congestion ☐ Coughing ☐ Chills ☐ Fever

Other symptoms: ______________________________

LET'S EXPLORE SOME MORE #39

Hours of Sleep	1	2	3	4	5	6	7	8	9	10	+
Sleep Quality	1	2	3	4	5	6	7	8	9	10	

WEATHER

- [ ] Hot
- [ ] Mild
- [ ] Cold
- [ ] Dry
- [ ] Humid
- [ ] Wet

BM Pressure: ______

Allergen Levels: ______

STRESS LEVELS

None	Low	Medium	High	Max	@$#%!

FOOD / MEDICATIONS

FOOD / DRINKS

MEDS / SUPPLEMENTS	TIME	DOSE

- [ ] usual daily medication

EXERCISE / DAILY ACTIVITY

- [ ] Heck yes, I worked out.
- [ ] I managed to exercise a bit.
- [ ] No, I haven't exercised at all.
- [ ] I did some stuff, and that counts.

DETAILS

NOTES / TRIGGERS / IMPROVEMENTS

WRITE ONE THING YOU'RE GRATEFUL FOR

Date:______________

HOW ARE YOU FEELING TODAY?

Like death

Terrible

Not good

Meh

Good

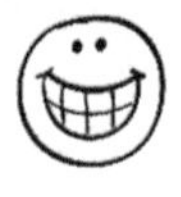
Great!

Amazing!

RATE YOUR PAIN LEVEL

1 2 3 4 5 6 7 8 9 10

Describe your pain / symptoms	am	pm
	☐	☐
	☐	☐
	☐	☐
	☐	☐
	☐	☐
	☐	☐
	☐	☐
	☐	☐

Where do you feel it?

Front *Back*

What about your...?

Mood	1	2	3	4	5	6	7	8	9	10
Energy levels	1	2	3	4	5	6	7	8	9	10
Mental clarity	1	2	3	4	5	6	7	8	9	10

Feeling sick?

☐ Nope!

☐ Yes...

☐ Nausea ☐ Diarrhea ☐ Vomiting ☐ Sore throat

☐ Congestion ☐ Coughing ☐ Chills ☐ Fever

Other symptoms: ____________________

LET'S EXPLORE SOME MORE

Hours of Sleep	1	2	3	4	5	6	7	8	9	10	+
Sleep Quality	1	2	3	4	5	6	7	8	9	10	

WEATHER

- ☐ Hot ☐ Mild ☐ Cold BM Pressure: ____
- ☐ Dry ☐ Humid ☐ Wet Allergen Levels: ____

STRESS LEVELS

None	Low	Medium	High	Max	@$#%!

FOOD / MEDICATIONS

FOOD / DRINKS

MEDS / SUPPLEMENTS	TIME	DOSE

☐ usual daily medication

EXERCISE / DAILY ACTIVITY

- ☐ Heck yes, I worked out.
- ☐ I managed to exercise a bit.
- ☐ No, I haven't exercised at all.
- ☐ I did some stuff, and that counts.

DETAILS

NOTES / TRIGGERS / IMPROVEMENTS

WRITE ONE THING YOU'RE GRATEFUL FOR

Date:______________

HOW ARE YOU FEELING TODAY?

Like death	Terrible	Not good	Meh	Good	Great!	Amazing!

RATE YOUR PAIN LEVEL

(1) (2) (3) (4) (5) (6) (7) (8) (9) (10)

Describe your pain / symptoms	am	pm
	☐	☐
	☐	☐
	☐	☐
	☐	☐
	☐	☐
	☐	☐
	☐	☐
	☐	☐

Where do you feel it?

Front *Back*

What about your...?

Mood	(1) (2) (3) (4) (5) (6) (7) (8) (9) (10)
Energy levels	(1) (2) (3) (4) (5) (6) (7) (8) (9) (10)
Mental clarity	(1) (2) (3) (4) (5) (6) (7) (8) (9) (10)

Feeling sick?

☐ Nope!
☐ Yes...

☐ Nausea	☐ Diarrhea	☐ Vomiting	☐ Sore throat
☐ Congestion	☐ Coughing	☐ Chills	☐ Fever

Other symptoms: ______________________________

LET'S EXPLORE SOME MORE

Hours of Sleep	1	2	3	4	5	6	7	8	9	10	+
Sleep Quality	1	2	3	4	5	6	7	8	9	10	

WEATHER

- ☐ Hot ☐ Mild ☐ Cold BM Pressure: ____
- ☐ Dry ☐ Humid ☐ Wet Allergen Levels: ____

STRESS LEVELS

None	Low	Medium	High	Max	@$#%!

FOOD / MEDICATIONS

FOOD / DRINKS

MEDS / SUPPLEMENTS	TIME	DOSE

☐ usual daily medication

EXERCISE / DAILY ACTIVITY

- ☐ Heck yes, I worked out.
- ☐ I managed to exercise a bit.
- ☐ No, I haven't exercised at all.
- ☐ I did some stuff, and that counts.

DETAILS

NOTES / TRIGGERS / IMPROVEMENTS

WRITE ONE THING YOU'RE GRATEFUL FOR

Date: ______________

HOW ARE YOU FEELING TODAY?

Like death | Terrible | Not good | Meh | Good | Great! | Amazing!

RATE YOUR PAIN LEVEL

① ② ③ ④ ⑤ ⑥ ⑦ ⑧ ⑨ ⑩

Describe your pain / symptoms	am	pm
	☐	☐
	☐	☐
	☐	☐
	☐	☐
	☐	☐
	☐	☐
	☐	☐
	☐	☐

Where do you feel it?

Front | *Back*

What about your...?

Mood	1	2	3	4	5	6	7	8	9	10
Energy levels	1	2	3	4	5	6	7	8	9	10
Mental clarity	1	2	3	4	5	6	7	8	9	10

Feeling sick?

☐ Nope!

☐ Yes...

☐ Nausea ☐ Diarrhea ☐ Vomiting ☐ Sore throat

☐ Congestion ☐ Coughing ☐ Chills ☐ Fever

Other symptoms: ______________________

LET'S EXPLORE SOME MORE

#42

Hours of Sleep	1	2	3	4	5	6	7	8	9	10	+
Sleep Quality	1	2	3	4	5	6	7	8	9	10	

WEATHER

- ☐ Hot ☐ Mild ☐ Cold BM Pressure: ____
- ☐ Dry ☐ Humid ☐ Wet Allergen Levels: ____

STRESS LEVELS

None	Low	Medium	High	Max	@$#%!

FOOD / MEDICATIONS

FOOD / DRINKS

MEDS / SUPPLEMENTS	TIME	DOSE

☐ usual daily medication

EXERCISE / DAILY ACTIVITY

- ☐ Heck yes, I worked out.
- ☐ I managed to exercise a bit.
- ☐ No, I haven't exercised at all.
- ☐ I did some stuff, and that counts.

DETAILS

NOTES / TRIGGERS / IMPROVEMENTS

WRITE ONE THING YOU'RE GRATEFUL FOR

Date: ______________

HOW ARE YOU FEELING TODAY?

Like death

Terrible

Not good

Meh

Good

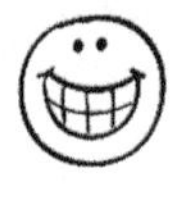
Great!

Amazing!

RATE YOUR PAIN LEVEL

① ② ③ ④ ⑤ ⑥ ⑦ ⑧ ⑨ ⑩

Describe your pain / symptoms	am	pm
	☐	☐
	☐	☐
	☐	☐
	☐	☐
	☐	☐
	☐	☐
	☐	☐
	☐	☐

Where do you feel it?

Front *Back*

What about your...?	
Mood	① ② ③ ④ ⑤ ⑥ ⑦ ⑧ ⑨ ⑩
Energy levels	① ② ③ ④ ⑤ ⑥ ⑦ ⑧ ⑨ ⑩
Mental clarity	① ② ③ ④ ⑤ ⑥ ⑦ ⑧ ⑨ ⑩

Feeling sick?

☐ Nope!

☐ Yes...

☐ Nausea	☐ Diarrhea	☐ Vomiting	☐ Sore throat
☐ Congestion	☐ Coughing	☐ Chills	☐ Fever

Other symptoms: ______________________________

LET'S EXPLORE SOME MORE #43

Hours of Sleep	1	2	3	4	5	6	7	8	9	10	+
Sleep Quality	1	2	3	4	5	6	7	8	9	10	

WEATHER

- ☐ Hot ☐ Mild ☐ Cold BM Pressure: ______
- ☐ Dry ☐ Humid ☐ Wet Allergen Levels: ______

STRESS LEVELS

None	Low	Medium	High	Max	@$#%!

FOOD / MEDICATIONS

FOOD / DRINKS

MEDS / SUPPLEMENTS	TIME	DOSE

☐ usual daily medication

EXERCISE / DAILY ACTIVITY

- ☐ Heck yes, I worked out.
- ☐ I managed to exercise a bit.
- ☐ No, I haven't exercised at all.
- ☐ I did some stuff, and that counts.

DETAILS

NOTES / TRIGGERS / IMPROVEMENTS

WRITE ONE THING YOU'RE GRATEFUL FOR

Date:____________

HOW ARE YOU FEELING TODAY?

Like death

Terrible

Not good

Meh

Good

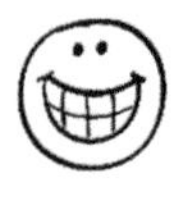
Great!

Amazing!

RATE YOUR PAIN LEVEL

① ② ③ ④ ⑤ ⑥ ⑦ ⑧ ⑨ ⑩

Describe your pain / symptoms	am	pm	Where do you feel it? Front	Back
	☐	☐		
	☐	☐		
	☐	☐		
	☐	☐		
	☐	☐		
	☐	☐		
	☐	☐		
	☐	☐		

What about your...?

Mood	① ② ③ ④ ⑤ ⑥ ⑦ ⑧ ⑨ ⑩	☐ Nope!
Energy levels	① ② ③ ④ ⑤ ⑥ ⑦ ⑧ ⑨ ⑩	☐ Yes...
Mental clarity	① ② ③ ④ ⑤ ⑥ ⑦ ⑧ ⑨ ⑩	

Feeling sick?

- ☐ Nausea
- ☐ Diarrhea
- ☐ Vomiting
- ☐ Sore throat
- ☐ Congestion
- ☐ Coughing
- ☐ Chills
- ☐ Fever

Other symptoms: ____________

LET'S EXPLORE SOME MORE #44

Hours of Sleep	(1) (2) (3) (4) (5) (6) (7) (8) (9) (10) (+)
Sleep Quality	(1) (2) (3) (4) (5) (6) (7) (8) (9) (10)

WEATHER

☐ Hot ☐ Mild ☐ Cold BM Pressure: ____

☐ Dry ☐ Humid ☐ Wet Allergen Levels: ____

STRESS LEVELS

None	Low	Medium	High	Max	@$#%!

FOOD / MEDICATIONS

FOOD / DRINKS

MEDS / SUPPLEMENTS	TIME	DOSE

☐ usual daily medication

EXERCISE / DAILY ACTIVITY

☐ Heck yes, I worked out.

☐ I managed to exercise a bit.

☐ No, I haven't exercised at all.

☐ I did some stuff, and that counts.

DETAILS

NOTES / TRIGGERS / IMPROVEMENTS

WRITE ONE THING YOU'RE GRATEFUL FOR

Date: ______________

HOW ARE YOU FEELING TODAY?

Like death	Terrible	Not good	Meh	Good	Great!	Amazing!

RATE YOUR PAIN LEVEL

① ② ③ ④ ⑤ ⑥ ⑦ ⑧ ⑨ ⑩

Describe your pain / symptoms	am	pm
	☐	☐
	☐	☐
	☐	☐
	☐	☐
	☐	☐
	☐	☐
	☐	☐
	☐	☐

Where do you feel it?

Front *Back*

What about your...?

Mood	1	2	3	4	5	6	7	8	9	10
Energy levels	1	2	3	4	5	6	7	8	9	10
Mental clarity	1	2	3	4	5	6	7	8	9	10

Feeling sick?

☐ Nope!

☐ Yes...

☐ Nausea ☐ Diarrhea ☐ Vomiting ☐ Sore throat

☐ Congestion ☐ Coughing ☐ Chills ☐ Fever

Other symptoms: ______________________

LET'S EXPLORE SOME MORE

Hours of Sleep	1 2 3 4 5 6 7 8 9 10 +
Sleep Quality	1 2 3 4 5 6 7 8 9 10

WEATHER

☐ Hot ☐ Mild ☐ Cold BM Pressure: ____

☐ Dry ☐ Humid ☐ Wet Allergen Levels: ____

STRESS LEVELS

None	Low	Medium	High	Max	@$#%!

FOOD / MEDICATIONS

FOOD / DRINKS

MEDS / SUPPLEMENTS	TIME	DOSE

☐ usual daily medication

EXERCISE / DAILY ACTIVITY

☐ Heck yes, I worked out.

☐ I managed to exercise a bit.

☐ No, I haven't exercised at all.

☐ I did some stuff, and that counts.

DETAILS

NOTES / TRIGGERS / IMPROVEMENTS

WRITE ONE THING YOU'RE GRATEFUL FOR

Date: ______________

HOW ARE YOU FEELING TODAY?

Like death	Terrible	Not good	Meh	Good	Great!	Amazing!

RATE YOUR PAIN LEVEL

(1) (2) (3) (4) (5) (6) (7) (8) (9) (10)

Describe your pain / symptoms	am	pm
	☐	☐
	☐	☐
	☐	☐
	☐	☐
	☐	☐
	☐	☐
	☐	☐
	☐	☐

Where do you feel it?

Front *Back*

What about your...?

Mood	(1) (2) (3) (4) (5) (6) (7) (8) (9) (10)
Energy levels	(1) (2) (3) (4) (5) (6) (7) (8) (9) (10)
Mental clarity	(1) (2) (3) (4) (5) (6) (7) (8) (9) (10)

Feeling sick?

☐ Nope!
☐ Yes...

☐ Nausea	☐ Diarrhea	☐ Vomiting	☐ Sore throat
☐ Congestion	☐ Coughing	☐ Chills	☐ Fever

Other symptoms: ______________________________

LET'S EXPLORE SOME MORE #46

Hours of Sleep	(1) (2) (3) (4) (5) (6) (7) (8) (9) (10) (+)
Sleep Quality	(1) (2) (3) (4) (5) (6) (7) (8) (9) (10)

WEATHER

☐ Hot ☐ Mild ☐ Cold BM Pressure: ______

☐ Dry ☐ Humid ☐ Wet Allergen Levels: ______

STRESS LEVELS

None	Low	Medium	High	Max	@$#%!

FOOD / MEDICATIONS

FOOD / DRINKS

MEDS / SUPPLEMENTS	TIME	DOSE

☐ usual daily medication

EXERCISE / DAILY ACTIVITY

☐ Heck yes, I worked out.

☐ I managed to exercise a bit.

☐ No, I haven't exercised at all.

☐ I did some stuff, and that counts.

DETAILS

NOTES / TRIGGERS / IMPROVEMENTS

WRITE ONE THING YOU'RE GRATEFUL FOR

Date: ______________

HOW ARE YOU FEELING TODAY?

Like death	Terrible	Not good	Meh	Good	Great!	Amazing!

RATE YOUR PAIN LEVEL

① ② ③ ④ ⑤ ⑥ ⑦ ⑧ ⑨ ⑩

Describe your pain / symptoms	am	pm
	☐	☐
	☐	☐
	☐	☐
	☐	☐
	☐	☐
	☐	☐
	☐	☐
	☐	☐

Where do you feel it?

Front *Back*

What about your...?

Mood	1	2	3	4	5	6	7	8	9	10
Energy levels	1	2	3	4	5	6	7	8	9	10
Mental clarity	1	2	3	4	5	6	7	8	9	10

Feeling sick?

☐ Nope!
☐ Yes...

☐ Nausea ☐ Diarrhea ☐ Vomiting ☐ Sore throat
☐ Congestion ☐ Coughing ☐ Chills ☐ Fever

Other symptoms: ______________________________

LET'S EXPLORE SOME MORE #47

Hours of Sleep	1	2	3	4	5	6	7	8	9	10	+
Sleep Quality	1	2	3	4	5	6	7	8	9	10	

WEATHER

- [ ] Hot
- [ ] Mild
- [ ] Cold

BM Pressure: ______

- [ ] Dry
- [ ] Humid
- [ ] Wet

Allergen Levels: ______

STRESS LEVELS

None	Low	Medium	High	Max	@$#%!

FOOD / MEDICATIONS

FOOD / DRINKS

MEDS / SUPPLEMENTS	TIME	DOSE

- [ ] usual daily medication

EXERCISE / DAILY ACTIVITY

- [ ] Heck yes, I worked out.
- [ ] I managed to exercise a bit.
- [ ] No, I haven't exercised at all.
- [ ] I did some stuff, and that counts.

DETAILS

NOTES / TRIGGERS / IMPROVEMENTS

WRITE ONE THING YOU'RE GRATEFUL FOR

Date: ______________

HOW ARE YOU FEELING TODAY?

Like death | Terrible | Not good | Meh | Good | Great! | Amazing!

RATE YOUR PAIN LEVEL

1 2 3 4 5 6 7 8 9 10

Describe your pain / symptoms	am	pm
	☐	☐
	☐	☐
	☐	☐
	☐	☐
	☐	☐
	☐	☐
	☐	☐
	☐	☐

Where do you feel it?

Front *Back*

What about your...?										
Mood	1	2	3	4	5	6	7	8	9	10
Energy levels	1	2	3	4	5	6	7	8	9	10
Mental clarity	1	2	3	4	5	6	7	8	9	10

Feeling sick?

☐ Nope!

☐ Yes...

☐ Nausea ☐ Diarrhea ☐ Vomiting ☐ Sore throat

☐ Congestion ☐ Coughing ☐ Chills ☐ Fever

Other symptoms: ______________________________

LET'S EXPLORE SOME MORE #48

Hours of Sleep	1 2 3 4 5 6 7 8 9 10 +
Sleep Quality	1 2 3 4 5 6 7 8 9 10

WEATHER

- [ ] Hot - [ ] Mild - [ ] Cold BM Pressure: ______
- [ ] Dry - [ ] Humid - [ ] Wet Allergen Levels: ______

STRESS LEVELS

None	Low	Medium	High	Max	@$#%!

FOOD / MEDICATIONS

FOOD / DRINKS

MEDS / SUPPLEMENTS	TIME	DOSE

- [ ] usual daily medication

EXERCISE / DAILY ACTIVITY

- [ ] Heck yes, I worked out.
- [ ] I managed to exercise a bit.
- [ ] No, I haven't exercised at all.
- [ ] I did some stuff, and that counts.

DETAILS

NOTES / TRIGGERS / IMPROVEMENTS

WRITE ONE THING YOU'RE GRATEFUL FOR

Date: _____________

HOW ARE YOU FEELING TODAY?

Like death	Terrible	Not good	Meh	Good	Great!	Amazing!

RATE YOUR PAIN LEVEL

① ② ③ ④ ⑤ ⑥ ⑦ ⑧ ⑨ ⑩

Describe your pain / symptoms	am	pm
	☐	☐
	☐	☐
	☐	☐
	☐	☐
	☐	☐
	☐	☐
	☐	☐
	☐	☐

Where do you feel it?

Front *Back*

What about your...?

Mood	1	2	3	4	5	6	7	8	9	10
Energy levels	1	2	3	4	5	6	7	8	9	10
Mental clarity	1	2	3	4	5	6	7	8	9	10

Feeling sick?

☐ Nope!

☐ Yes...

☐ Nausea	☐ Diarrhea	☐ Vomiting	☐ Sore throat
☐ Congestion	☐ Coughing	☐ Chills	☐ Fever

Other symptoms: ____________________

LET'S EXPLORE SOME MORE

#49

Hours of Sleep	(1) (2) (3) (4) (5) (6) (7) (8) (9) (10) (+)
Sleep Quality	(1) (2) (3) (4) (5) (6) (7) (8) (9) (10)

WEATHER

☐ Hot	☐ Mild	☐ Cold	BM Pressure: ______
☐ Dry	☐ Humid	☐ Wet	Allergen Levels: ______

STRESS LEVELS

None	Low	Medium	High	Max	@$#%!

FOOD / MEDICATIONS

FOOD / DRINKS

MEDS / SUPPLEMENTS	TIME	DOSE

☐ usual daily medication

EXERCISE / DAILY ACTIVITY

- ☐ Heck yes, I worked out.
- ☐ I managed to exercise a bit.
- ☐ No, I haven't exercised at all.
- ☐ I did some stuff, and that counts.

DETAILS

NOTES / TRIGGERS / IMPROVEMENTS

WRITE ONE THING YOU'RE GRATEFUL FOR

Date:______________

HOW ARE YOU FEELING TODAY?

Like death

Terrible

Not good

Meh

Good

Great!

Amazing!

RATE YOUR PAIN LEVEL

1 2 3 4 5 6 7 8 9 10

Describe your pain / symptoms	am	pm	Where do you feel it? Front	Back
	☐	☐		
	☐	☐		
	☐	☐		
	☐	☐		
	☐	☐		
	☐	☐		
	☐	☐		
	☐	☐		

What about your...?		Feeling sick?
Mood	1 2 3 4 5 6 7 8 9 10	☐ Nope!
Energy levels	1 2 3 4 5 6 7 8 9 10	☐ Yes...
Mental clarity	1 2 3 4 5 6 7 8 9 10	

☐ Nausea ☐ Diarrhea ☐ Vomiting ☐ Sore throat
☐ Congestion ☐ Coughing ☐ Chills ☐ Fever

Other symptoms: ____________________

LET'S EXPLORE SOME MORE #50

Hours of Sleep	1 2 3 4 5 6 7 8 9 10 +
Sleep Quality	1 2 3 4 5 6 7 8 9 10

WEATHER

- ☐ Hot ☐ Mild ☐ Cold BM Pressure: ____
- ☐ Dry ☐ Humid ☐ Wet Allergen Levels: ____

STRESS LEVELS

None	Low	Medium	High	Max	@$#%!

FOOD / MEDICATIONS

FOOD / DRINKS

MEDS / SUPPLEMENTS	TIME	DOSE

☐ usual daily medication

EXERCISE / DAILY ACTIVITY

- ☐ Heck yes, I worked out.
- ☐ I managed to exercise a bit.
- ☐ No, I haven't exercised at all.
- ☐ I did some stuff, and that counts.

DETAILS

NOTES / TRIGGERS / IMPROVEMENTS

WRITE ONE THING YOU'RE GRATEFUL FOR

Date: ______________

HOW ARE YOU FEELING TODAY?

Like death	Terrible	Not good	Meh	Good	Great!	Amazing!

RATE YOUR PAIN LEVEL

① ② ③ ④ ⑤ ⑥ ⑦ ⑧ ⑨ ⑩

Describe your pain / symptoms	am	pm
	☐	☐
	☐	☐
	☐	☐
	☐	☐
	☐	☐
	☐	☐
	☐	☐
	☐	☐

Where do you feel it?

Front *Back*

What about your...?

Mood	1	2	3	4	5	6	7	8	9	10
Energy levels	1	2	3	4	5	6	7	8	9	10
Mental clarity	1	2	3	4	5	6	7	8	9	10

Feeling sick?

☐ Nope!
☐ Yes...

☐ Nausea ☐ Diarrhea ☐ Vomiting ☐ Sore throat
☐ Congestion ☐ Coughing ☐ Chills ☐ Fever

Other symptoms: ______________________________

LET'S EXPLORE SOME MORE

#51

Hours of Sleep	1	2	3	4	5	6	7	8	9	10	+
Sleep Quality	1	2	3	4	5	6	7	8	9	10	

WEATHER

- [ ] Hot
- [ ] Mild
- [ ] Cold

BM Pressure: ______

- [ ] Dry
- [ ] Humid
- [ ] Wet

Allergen Levels: ______

STRESS LEVELS

None	Low	Medium	High	Max	@$#%!

FOOD / MEDICATIONS

FOOD / DRINKS

MEDS / SUPPLEMENTS	TIME	DOSE

- [ ] usual daily medication

EXERCISE / DAILY ACTIVITY

- [ ] Heck yes, I worked out.
- [ ] I managed to exercise a bit.
- [ ] No, I haven't exercised at all.
- [ ] I did some stuff, and that counts.

DETAILS

NOTES / TRIGGERS / IMPROVEMENTS

WRITE ONE THING YOU'RE GRATEFUL FOR

Date: ______________

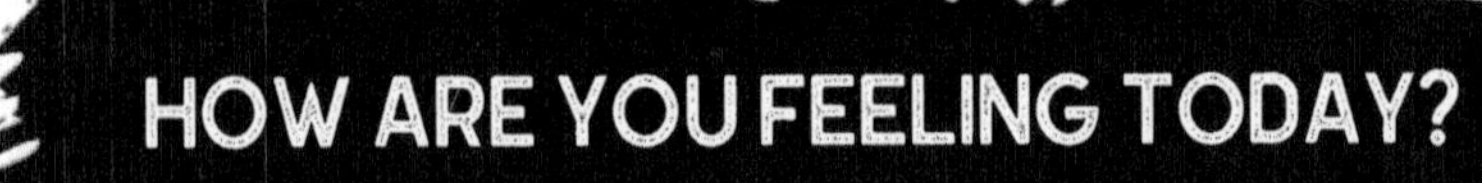

					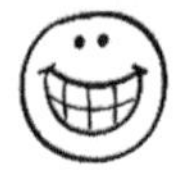	
Like death	Terrible	Not good	Meh	Good	Great!	Amazing!

RATE YOUR PAIN LEVEL

① ② ③ ④ ⑤ ⑥ ⑦ ⑧ ⑨ ⑩

Describe your pain / symptoms	am	pm
	☐	☐
	☐	☐
	☐	☐
	☐	☐
	☐	☐
	☐	☐
	☐	☐
	☐	☐

Where do you feel it?

Front *Back*

What about your...?

Mood	① ② ③ ④ ⑤ ⑥ ⑦ ⑧ ⑨ ⑩
Energy levels	① ② ③ ④ ⑤ ⑥ ⑦ ⑧ ⑨ ⑩
Mental clarity	① ② ③ ④ ⑤ ⑥ ⑦ ⑧ ⑨ ⑩

Feeling sick?

☐ Nope!

☐ Yes...

☐ Nausea	☐ Diarrhea	☐ Vomiting	☐ Sore throat
☐ Congestion	☐ Coughing	☐ Chills	☐ Fever

Other symptoms: ______________________________

LET'S EXPLORE SOME MORE

Hours of Sleep	① ② ③ ④ ⑤ ⑥ ⑦ ⑧ ⑨ ⑩ (+)
Sleep Quality	① ② ③ ④ ⑤ ⑥ ⑦ ⑧ ⑨ ⑩

WEATHER

☐ Hot ☐ Mild ☐ Cold BM Pressure: ____

☐ Dry ☐ Humid ☐ Wet Allergen Levels: ____

STRESS LEVELS

None	Low	Medium	High	Max	@$#%!

FOOD / MEDICATIONS

FOOD / DRINKS

MEDS / SUPPLEMENTS	TIME	DOSE

☐ usual daily medication

EXERCISE / DAILY ACTIVITY

☐ Heck yes, I worked out.

☐ I managed to exercise a bit.

☐ No, I haven't exercised at all.

☐ I did some stuff, and that counts.

DETAILS

NOTES / TRIGGERS / IMPROVEMENTS

WRITE ONE THING YOU'RE GRATEFUL FOR

Date: _______________

HOW ARE YOU FEELING TODAY?

     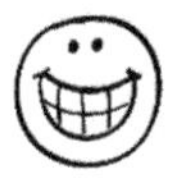 

Like death	Terrible	Not good	Meh	Good	Great!	Amazing!

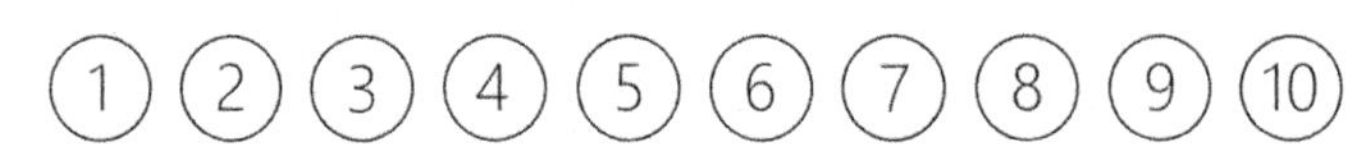

RATE YOUR PAIN LEVEL

1 2 3 4 5 6 7 8 9 10

Describe your pain / symptoms	am	pm
	☐	☐
	☐	☐
	☐	☐
	☐	☐
	☐	☐
	☐	☐
	☐	☐
	☐	☐

Where do you feel it?

Front *Back*

What about your...?

Mood	1 2 3 4 5 6 7 8 9 10
Energy levels	1 2 3 4 5 6 7 8 9 10
Mental clarity	1 2 3 4 5 6 7 8 9 10

Feeling sick?

☐ Nope!
☐ Yes...

☐ Nausea	☐ Diarrhea	☐ Vomiting	☐ Sore throat
☐ Congestion	☐ Coughing	☐ Chills	☐ Fever

Other symptoms: ____________________

LET'S EXPLORE SOME MORE

Hours of Sleep	1 2 3 4 5 6 7 8 9 10 +
Sleep Quality	1 2 3 4 5 6 7 8 9 10

WEATHER

- ☐ Hot ☐ Mild ☐ Cold BM Pressure: ____
- ☐ Dry ☐ Humid ☐ Wet Allergen Levels: ____

STRESS LEVELS

None	Low	Medium	High	Max	@$#%!

FOOD / MEDICATIONS

FOOD / DRINKS

MEDS / SUPPLEMENTS	TIME	DOSE

☐ usual daily medication

EXERCISE / DAILY ACTIVITY

- ☐ Heck yes, I worked out.
- ☐ I managed to exercise a bit.
- ☐ No, I haven't exercised at all.
- ☐ I did some stuff, and that counts.

DETAILS

NOTES / TRIGGERS / IMPROVEMENTS

WRITE ONE THING YOU'RE GRATEFUL FOR

Date: ______________

HOW ARE YOU FEELING TODAY?

Like death

Terrible

Not good

Meh

Good

Great!

Amazing!

RATE YOUR PAIN LEVEL

① ② ③ ④ ⑤ ⑥ ⑦ ⑧ ⑨ ⑩

Describe your pain / symptoms	am	pm
	☐	☐
	☐	☐
	☐	☐
	☐	☐
	☐	☐
	☐	☐
	☐	☐
	☐	☐

Where do you feel it?

Front *Back*

What about your...?

Mood	1	2	3	4	5	6	7	8	9	10
Energy levels	1	2	3	4	5	6	7	8	9	10
Mental clarity	1	2	3	4	5	6	7	8	9	10

Feeling sick?

- ☐ Nope!
- ☐ Yes...

☐ Nausea	☐ Diarrhea	☐ Vomiting	☐ Sore throat
☐ Congestion	☐ Coughing	☐ Chills	☐ Fever

Other symptoms: ______________________

LET'S EXPLORE SOME MORE

#54

Hours of Sleep	1	2	3	4	5	6	7	8	9	10	+
Sleep Quality	1	2	3	4	5	6	7	8	9	10	

WEATHER

- [ ] Hot
- [ ] Mild
- [ ] Cold
- [ ] Dry
- [ ] Humid
- [ ] Wet

BM Pressure: ______

Allergen Levels: ______

STRESS LEVELS

None	Low	Medium	High	Max	@$#%!

FOOD / MEDICATIONS

FOOD / DRINKS

MEDS / SUPPLEMENTS	TIME	DOSE

- [ ] usual daily medication

EXERCISE / DAILY ACTIVITY

- [ ] Heck yes, I worked out.
- [ ] I managed to exercise a bit.
- [ ] No, I haven't exercised at all.
- [ ] I did some stuff, and that counts.

DETAILS

NOTES / TRIGGERS / IMPROVEMENTS

WRITE ONE THING YOU'RE GRATEFUL FOR

Date:______________

HOW ARE YOU FEELING TODAY?

Like death	Terrible	Not good	Meh	Good	Great!	Amazing!

RATE YOUR PAIN LEVEL

① ② ③ ④ ⑤ ⑥ ⑦ ⑧ ⑨ ⑩

Describe your pain / symptoms	am	pm	Where do you feel it? Front	Back
	☐	☐		
	☐	☐		
	☐	☐		
	☐	☐		
	☐	☐		
	☐	☐		
	☐	☐		
	☐	☐		

What about your...?

Mood	1	2	3	4	5	6	7	8	9	10
Energy levels	1	2	3	4	5	6	7	8	9	10
Mental clarity	1	2	3	4	5	6	7	8	9	10

Feeling sick?

☐ Nope!

☐ Yes...

☐ Nausea ☐ Diarrhea ☐ Vomiting ☐ Sore throat

☐ Congestion ☐ Coughing ☐ Chills ☐ Fever

Other symptoms: ______________________

LET'S EXPLORE SOME MORE

Hours of Sleep	1	2	3	4	5	6	7	8	9	10	+
Sleep Quality	1	2	3	4	5	6	7	8	9	10	

WEATHER

☐ Hot ☐ Mild ☐ Cold BM Pressure: ______

☐ Dry ☐ Humid ☐ Wet Allergen Levels: ______

STRESS LEVELS

None	Low	Medium	High	Max	@$#%!

FOOD / MEDICATIONS

FOOD / DRINKS

MEDS / SUPPLEMENTS	TIME	DOSE

☐ usual daily medication

EXERCISE / DAILY ACTIVITY

☐ Heck yes, I worked out.

☐ I managed to exercise a bit.

☐ No, I haven't exercised at all.

☐ I did some stuff, and that counts.

DETAILS

NOTES / TRIGGERS / IMPROVEMENTS

WRITE ONE THING YOU'RE GRATEFUL FOR

Date: ______________

HOW ARE YOU FEELING TODAY?

Like death

Terrible

Not good

Meh

Good

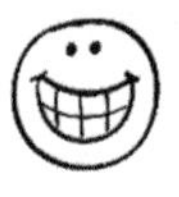
Great!

Amazing!

RATE YOUR PAIN LEVEL

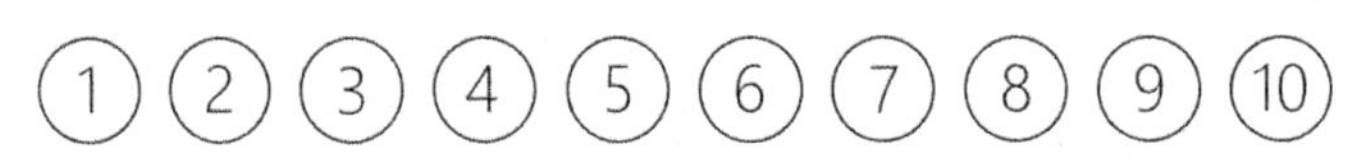

Describe your pain / symptoms	am	pm
	☐	☐
	☐	☐
	☐	☐
	☐	☐
	☐	☐
	☐	☐
	☐	☐
	☐	☐

Where do you feel it?

Front *Back*

What about your...?										
Mood	1	2	3	4	5	6	7	8	9	10
Energy levels	1	2	3	4	5	6	7	8	9	10
Mental clarity	1	2	3	4	5	6	7	8	9	10

Feeling sick?

☐ Nope!

☐ Yes...

☐ Nausea	☐ Diarrhea	☐ Vomiting	☐ Sore throat
☐ Congestion	☐ Coughing	☐ Chills	☐ Fever

Other symptoms: ______________________________

LET'S EXPLORE SOME MORE

Hours of Sleep	1	2	3	4	5	6	7	8	9	10	+
Sleep Quality	1	2	3	4	5	6	7	8	9	10	

WEATHER

- [ ] Hot
- [ ] Mild
- [ ] Cold
- [ ] Dry
- [ ] Humid
- [ ] Wet

BM Pressure: ______

Allergen Levels: ______

STRESS LEVELS

None	Low	Medium	High	Max	@$#%!

FOOD / MEDICATIONS

FOOD / DRINKS

MEDS / SUPPLEMENTS	TIME	DOSE

- [ ] usual daily medication

EXERCISE / DAILY ACTIVITY

- [ ] Heck yes, I worked out.
- [ ] I managed to exercise a bit.
- [ ] No, I haven't exercised at all.
- [ ] I did some stuff, and that counts.

DETAILS

NOTES / TRIGGERS / IMPROVEMENTS

WRITE ONE THING YOU'RE GRATEFUL FOR

Date: ______________

HOW ARE YOU FEELING TODAY?

Like death | Terrible | Not good | Meh | Good | Great! | Amazing!

RATE YOUR PAIN LEVEL

① ② ③ ④ ⑤ ⑥ ⑦ ⑧ ⑨ ⑩

Describe your pain / symptoms	am	pm
	☐	☐
	☐	☐
	☐	☐
	☐	☐
	☐	☐
	☐	☐
	☐	☐
	☐	☐

Where do you feel it?

Front | *Back*

What about your...?

Mood	① ② ③ ④ ⑤ ⑥ ⑦ ⑧ ⑨ ⑩
Energy levels	① ② ③ ④ ⑤ ⑥ ⑦ ⑧ ⑨ ⑩
Mental clarity	① ② ③ ④ ⑤ ⑥ ⑦ ⑧ ⑨ ⑩

Feeling sick?

☐ Nope!

☐ Yes...

☐ Nausea ☐ Diarrhea ☐ Vomiting ☐ Sore throat

☐ Congestion ☐ Coughing ☐ Chills ☐ Fever

Other symptoms: ______________________________

LET'S EXPLORE SOME MORE

#57

Hours of Sleep	1	2	3	4	5	6	7	8	9	10	+
Sleep Quality	1	2	3	4	5	6	7	8	9	10	

WEATHER

- [ ] Hot
- [ ] Mild
- [ ] Cold
- [ ] Dry
- [ ] Humid
- [ ] Wet

BM Pressure: ____

Allergen Levels: ____

STRESS LEVELS

None	Low	Medium	High	Max	@$#%!

FOOD / MEDICATIONS

FOOD / DRINKS

MEDS / SUPPLEMENTS	TIME	DOSE

- [ ] usual daily medication

EXERCISE / DAILY ACTIVITY

- [ ] Heck yes, I worked out.
- [ ] I managed to exercise a bit.
- [ ] No, I haven't exercised at all.
- [ ] I did some stuff, and that counts.

DETAILS

NOTES / TRIGGERS / IMPROVEMENTS

WRITE ONE THING YOU'RE GRATEFUL FOR

Date: _______________

HOW ARE YOU FEELING TODAY?

Like death

Terrible

Not good

Meh

Good

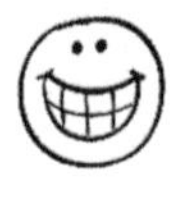
Great!

Amazing!

RATE YOUR PAIN LEVEL

① ② ③ ④ ⑤ ⑥ ⑦ ⑧ ⑨ ⑩

Describe your pain / symptoms	am	pm	Where do you feel it? Front	Back
	☐	☐		
	☐	☐		
	☐	☐		
	☐	☐		
	☐	☐		
	☐	☐		
	☐	☐		
	☐	☐		

What about your...?		Feeling sick?
Mood	① ② ③ ④ ⑤ ⑥ ⑦ ⑧ ⑨ ⑩	☐ Nope!
Energy levels	① ② ③ ④ ⑤ ⑥ ⑦ ⑧ ⑨ ⑩	☐ Yes...
Mental clarity	① ② ③ ④ ⑤ ⑥ ⑦ ⑧ ⑨ ⑩	

☐ Nausea ☐ Diarrhea ☐ Vomiting ☐ Sore throat

☐ Congestion ☐ Coughing ☐ Chills ☐ Fever

Other symptoms: _______________

LET'S EXPLORE SOME MORE

Hours of Sleep	1	2	3	4	5	6	7	8	9	10	+
Sleep Quality	1	2	3	4	5	6	7	8	9	10	

WEATHER

- [ ] Hot
- [ ] Mild
- [ ] Cold
- [ ] Dry
- [ ] Humid
- [ ] Wet

BM Pressure: ______

Allergen Levels: ______

STRESS LEVELS

None	Low	Medium	High	Max	@$#%!

FOOD / MEDICATIONS

FOOD / DRINKS

MEDS / SUPPLEMENTS	TIME	DOSE

- [ ] usual daily medication

EXERCISE / DAILY ACTIVITY

- [ ] Heck yes, I worked out.
- [ ] I managed to exercise a bit.
- [ ] No, I haven't exercised at all.
- [ ] I did some stuff, and that counts.

DETAILS

NOTES / TRIGGERS / IMPROVEMENTS

WRITE ONE THING YOU'RE GRATEFUL FOR

Date: ______________

HOW ARE YOU FEELING TODAY?

Like death	Terrible	Not good	Meh	Good	Great!	Amazing!

RATE YOUR PAIN LEVEL

1 2 3 4 5 6 7 8 9 10

Describe your pain / symptoms	am	pm	Where do you feel it? Front	Back
	☐	☐		
	☐	☐		
	☐	☐		
	☐	☐		
	☐	☐		
	☐	☐		
	☐	☐		
	☐	☐		

What about your...?		Feeling sick?
Mood	1 2 3 4 5 6 7 8 9 10	☐ Nope!
Energy levels	1 2 3 4 5 6 7 8 9 10	☐ Yes...
Mental clarity	1 2 3 4 5 6 7 8 9 10	

☐ Nausea	☐ Diarrhea	☐ Vomiting	☐ Sore throat
☐ Congestion	☐ Coughing	☐ Chills	☐ Fever

Other symptoms: ______________________________

LET'S EXPLORE SOME MORE #59

Hours of Sleep	1	2	3	4	5	6	7	8	9	10	+
Sleep Quality	1	2	3	4	5	6	7	8	9	10	

WEATHER

- ☐ Hot ☐ Mild ☐ Cold BM Pressure: ______
- ☐ Dry ☐ Humid ☐ Wet Allergen Levels: ______

STRESS LEVELS

None	Low	Medium	High	Max	@$#%!

FOOD / MEDICATIONS

FOOD / DRINKS

MEDS / SUPPLEMENTS	TIME	DOSE

☐ usual daily medication

EXERCISE / DAILY ACTIVITY

- ☐ Heck yes, I worked out.
- ☐ I managed to exercise a bit.
- ☐ No, I haven't exercised at all.
- ☐ I did some stuff, and that counts.

DETAILS

NOTES / TRIGGERS / IMPROVEMENTS

WRITE ONE THING YOU'RE GRATEFUL FOR

Date: ______________

HOW ARE YOU FEELING TODAY?

Like death	Terrible	Not good	Meh	Good	Great!	Amazing!

RATE YOUR PAIN LEVEL

(1) (2) (3) (4) (5) (6) (7) (8) (9) (10)

Describe your pain / symptoms | Where do you feel it?

	am	pm
	☐	☐
	☐	☐
	☐	☐
	☐	☐
	☐	☐
	☐	☐
	☐	☐
	☐	☐

Front *Back*

What about your...? | Feeling sick?

Mood	(1) (2) (3) (4) (5) (6) (7) (8) (9) (10)
Energy levels	(1) (2) (3) (4) (5) (6) (7) (8) (9) (10)
Mental clarity	(1) (2) (3) (4) (5) (6) (7) (8) (9) (10)

☐ Nope!
☐ Yes...

☐ Nausea	☐ Diarrhea	☐ Vomiting	☐ Sore throat
☐ Congestion	☐ Coughing	☐ Chills	☐ Fever

Other symptoms: ______________________

LET'S EXPLORE SOME MORE

#60

Hours of Sleep	1	2	3	4	5	6	7	8	9	10	+
Sleep Quality	1	2	3	4	5	6	7	8	9	10	

WEATHER

- [ ] Hot
- [ ] Mild
- [ ] Cold
- [ ] Dry
- [ ] Humid
- [ ] Wet

BM Pressure: ______

Allergen Levels: ______

STRESS LEVELS

None	Low	Medium	High	Max	@$#%!

FOOD / MEDICATIONS

FOOD / DRINKS

MEDS / SUPPLEMENTS	TIME	DOSE

- [ ] usual daily medication

EXERCISE / DAILY ACTIVITY

- [ ] Heck yes, I worked out.
- [ ] I managed to exercise a bit.
- [ ] No, I haven't exercised at all.
- [ ] I did some stuff, and that counts.

DETAILS

NOTES / TRIGGERS / IMPROVEMENTS

WRITE ONE THING YOU'RE GRATEFUL FOR

NOTES

Printed in Great Britain
by Amazon